AMANDA TATTAM is a journalist who has written for numerous newspapers and magazines in Australia and overseas. She is the editor of *From the Heart: True stories by Australian nurses* and *Tales from the Blackboard: True stories by Australian teachers*. She is also a registered nurse.

CATE KENNEDY is a short story author and poet whose work has won several national awards, including the *Age* Short Story Award and the Vincent Buckley Poetry Prize. She works as a writer-in-residence in schools around Victoria and teaches creative writing through the Victorian Writers' Centre.

LABOUR of LOVE

TALES FROM THE WORLD OF MIDWIVES

Edited by
AMANDA TATTAM & CATE KENNEDY

Cate Kennedy

PAN
Pan Macmillan Australia

First published 2005 in Pan by Pan Macmillan Australia Pty Limited
St Martins Tower, 31 Market Street, Sydney

National Library of Australia
Cataloguing-in-Publication data

Labour of love : tales from the world of midwives.

ISBN 0 330 42166 2.

1. Midwives - Australia - Anecdotes. 2. Childbirth - Australia.
I. Tattam, Amanda. II. Kennedy, Cate.

618.20231

Papers used by Pan Macmillan Australia Pty Ltd are natural, recyclable products made from wood grown in sustainable forests. The manufacturing processes conform to the environmental regulations of the country of origin.

Set in 11 pt Sabon by Midland Typesetters
Printed in Australia by McPherson's Printing Group

CONTENTS

FOREWORD

PROFESSOR FIONA STANLEY AC, AUSTRALIAN OF THE YEAR 2003

There are precious few times in life when you are fortunate enough to meet people who bring you a truly new perspective on a subject that you thought you knew – people who inspire you to ask different questions and re-evaluate the essence of what you're doing.

Certainly that was my experience when I first began working with midwives, and it is why I am so deeply honoured to write the foreword to this wonderful collection of stories.

My relationship with midwives began when I first branched out into maternal and child health research. Indeed my very first research assistant back in 1977 was a midwife – Barbara Chester. What was so apparent about Barbara and her colleagues was that they, as midwives, understood the importance of asking the questions about why things sometimes go wrong – birth defects, what precedes premature birth, low birth weight, cerebral palsy, stillbirth and so on. They understood that these outcomes were more than just medical issues to be tackled; they profoundly affected individual children and families. That it wasn't simply medical interventions that we should strive for, but a better understanding of how to prevent these things from happening at all.

I guess you could say that's why midwives and I have such a strong bond. I came from medical training, where people were always trying to outsmart each other. The midwives I worked with didn't have that sort of ego – their focus was on that particular mother, her baby and everything that was important for the future of that family. I think a major difference between doctors and midwives is that midwives are trained to care – trained to put their patient in the middle and work around their needs. Midwives knew that the questions the research team wanted to ask would help some families understand what had happened to them, and help prevent other families from experiencing the same trauma. It was personal.

So for me it was a real turning point to meet up with a group of women (as it was in those days) prepared to commit their scientific and practical knowledge to improving outcomes for mothers, babies and families. That knowledge became the essence of the Western Australian Midwives Notification System, a groundbreaking database we set up in the 1970s that has recorded information about every birth in WA since that time. It's relied upon a wonderful commitment from every midwife to provide perinatal information about every birth. For researchers like me, it's pure gold; internationally, it's considered to be the very best data set of its kind. The information has been absolutely crucial to our understanding of prematurity, the impact of interventions, and to describing the antenatal and perinatal contributions to cerebral palsy, childhood illnesses and growth and development. I know that many more answers will still be found in that treasure trove of data.

Midwives have also been important members of the research team in specific projects set up to investigate the prevention of pre-term birth, birth defects, cerebral palsy, the rate of caesarean sections and the issues around homebirths. To all these studies they brought more than their professional skills; they provided a different perspective. They had their own questions to add – different ones to mine – based on their own experiences. They asked some of the same questions, but in a different way, broadening the value of the projects immensely.

Fundamentally, what they brought was a more holistic approach, and it's that approach that has influenced me tremendously and how I now see research. It is a constant reminder to always think of what the data means for the mother, the baby, the family – and how it will improve their care and their lives.

Reading the stories in this book has brought me both laughter and tears. The tales from the bedside reveal both the joys and devastation that can accompany birth, and how that touches the lives of the midwives who are both facilitators and witnesses to it all. It is true that people don't really understand what midwives do – perhaps that in itself is a reflection of their professionalism as they quietly touch a family's life in the most precious of moments. I'm sure you will enjoy reading this book as much as I did. It is a powerful tribute to all midwives – many of whom I am proud to count as fine colleagues and friends.

Through the eyes of midwives

AMANDA TATTAM &
CATE KENNEDY

In the time it takes you to read this introduction, many hundreds of women in Australia will have been coaxed, soothed, touched and reassured by a midwife.

While birth and caring for babies is far from predictable, the care and attention of midwives is one of the crucial comforts for labouring women and their families, whether they are welcoming new life into the world in hospitals or homes, in birthing centres, in baths or – unexpectedly – on front verandahs. Yet midwives are almost invisible in literature and in public life.

The title of one of the stories in this collection states this baldly: 'People don't know what we do.' That story isn't a whinge about professional marginalisation. It is a tenderly told account of the invisible work undertaken to help people devastated by grief. In it, midwives care for a premature baby who has died and prepare a memento for her parents. '"A 23-weeker," says Gabi. "I've washed and dressed her. Now I'm doing the album for the parents." She pulls a booklet from the shelf under the cot and opens it to the first page.'

People don't see this labour of love. It goes on behind the scenes, like so much 'women's work' – unseen and unacknowledged, away from 'The trumpets and the cavalry' described in the story by Nola Aicken.

Obstetricians are nearly always the public face of maternity services. Confident and independent, they are not beholden to a hospital hierarchy that demands loyalty and obedience from its workforce. Doctors are seen as leaders in the 'maternity world', and despite all the advances of feminism and equal opportunity in the workplace, midwives are subordinate – yet eternally devoted. It is this hidden and emotionally gruelling world that is now being aired by a profession that is frustratingly seen as a 'branch' of nursing or as assistants or adjuncts to doctors.

Across cultures, though, and across history, midwives are there, and have always been there. Conception, birth and the traditional rituals of childbearing have historically been surrounded by mystique, and the unknown induces fear. The often closely guarded skills of midwives have seen them throughout history both persecuted as witches and respected as sages. In fact, the ancient Jews called midwives 'wise women' and the phrase has remained intact in several languages: *sage femme* in French, for example, and *weise frau* in German. In some

African cultures, the word 'midwife' is synonymous with 'spiritual healer'.

The stories in this collection are often graphically candid, because there aren't many secrets midwives aren't privy to. They are witnesses to profoundly emotional moments; highly skilled practitioners who regularly have to negotiate complex clinical situations and make life or death decisions for mothers and babies. You may have gripped their hand as you gave birth, or wept on their shoulder, or confided in them your most intimate private fears, yet who really understands the intricacies of their work and the value of their contribution to the healthcare system?

Aren't they just the same as nurses?

Each year there are around 252,000 babies born in Australia – that's 690 every day, or 29 every hour – and it's more than likely that at least one midwife will be there, nurturing women, men and others in the birth circle.

But that's not the only work of midwives. Their presence is felt in many other settings – caring for those trying to conceive, pregnant women, those giving birth, or in the postnatal period, or in neonatal intensive care units and well into the baby's first year of life. Indeed, the majority of early childhood/maternal and child health nurses are also midwives. From the outset we have wanted to strip back the notion that midwives only work in acute settings and ensure that the voices of maternal and child health nurses are heard very clearly.

Rewarding as the work is in nurturing those quarter of a million new Australians into the world every year, the midwifery profession is facing a crisis. By 2012, it is estimated there will be a shortfall of 1850 midwives in Australia.[1] Would you like to be having a baby then? In some cases new graduates are quitting the profession at a rate faster than older midwives are retiring. There is widespread disillusionment about an inability to practise autonomously; about rising levels of technical intervention in birth, about an endemic fear of litigation, and about the lack of resources available to provide genuine woman-centred care. All of this is changing traditional birthing choices irrevocably.

The desire to address the invisibility of midwives and to write about their work originated in 2002, when the North Central Victorian branch of the Australian College of Midwives Inc. (ACMI) called on its members and colleagues to write narrative accounts of their experiences for a local competition. In 2003, this enthusiastic group of midwives – Marie Treloar, Nola Aicken, Helen Sandner, Marg Rinaldi and Fran Sheehan – decided, with our help, to broaden the competition to include anyone in Australia who has worked as a midwife or maternal and child health nurse. The group approached us to help organise and judge the competition, called Midwives, Miracles and Mayhem (MMM). As there are only 11,985 practising midwives in Australia (8754 full timers) – a small number compared with nurses and teachers – it was always going to be difficult to elicit a big response. The winning stories were 'Birth in a parallel universe' (first prize), 'Broken waters' (second prize) and 'Breakfast at Simone's' (third prize). After the competition we commissioned more stories via ACMI networks, conferences, word of mouth and writers' centres in each state and territory. It seems there are more retired midwives, or people with a midwifery qualification who no longer practise, than there are those still doing clinical work.

The aims of the MMM project were:

- to explore the experiences of midwives at work in Australia in many different settings – antenatal/postnatal/community midwifery centres/regional and remote areas/homebirthing and caring for babies and mothers after they come home
- to educate and entertain the community about the valuable and often misunderstood role of midwives
- to highlight the shortage of qualified and experienced midwives and inspire the next generation of young people to join the profession
- to give voice to new and emerging writers who wish to share their personal experiences for their own personal and professional growth.

In this book, we present the sometimes polarised emotional world of midwives. Take this description by Shannon Morris:

> The baby started to turn to face me, but the doctor decided she might want to go the other way! Luckily she just kept coming, but not before another set of hands came out of the blue to get in on the action, pulling and shoving. This baby wasn't so much born as yanked from her mother's body. All blue and floppy, I guided her up to her mother's breast. The placenta was born. Maryanne had a bit of a tear – was that us? They assure me not.
>
> It was special to feel a newborn slide through my hands, so why, then, did I get in my car at the end of the day and cry?

Midwives, like the nurses who wrote their stories for *From the Heart: True stories by Australian nurses*[2] often carry an enormous load of grief with them. We expect them to store this somewhere, and to get on with the job at hand. It's not often they have the opportunity to debrief after traumatic or memorable events. Some of the events described in this book happened many years ago, and the midwives who wrote them told us they still wept on recalling them.

The stories straddle many decades; some are set in the 1950s and 1960s, others are contemporary, and, viewed together, they are testament to changes in policy and social stigma, to ideas about appropriate care, and to the shifting complexities of working across cultures. We hear midwives, for example, writing about adoption from their perspective. Dianne Boshammer writes about a baby she cared for who had a profound effect on all those who looked after her:

> Nearly twenty years on, I still think of Sarah. I ask myself: why did this little baby have such an impact on me? Was it my age and circumstances? I was married yet childless, and just starting to think about having a family. Was it the timing of Sarah's birth during my midwifery training, and the experiences I gained looking after her? What was it about her?

We hear about a time when a maternal and child health nurse was able to take a crying baby home for a weekend when the parents were at their wits' end. We hear of a midwife frantically ringing around Australia for interpreters as a Somalian woman lies in labour, alone and unable to communicate with anyone. We read of ingenious, unorthodox techniques which hasten delivery, save lives, and solve breastfeeding dilemmas. We laugh in commiseration as Brooke McReynolds gamely tries to incorporate new fashions into her practice:

> Mum was seated on the birthing stool near the end of the bed, close enough to lean over the mattress if she wanted to. She, the CTG machine (baby monitor) and the bedside table piled high with drinks, munchies, and massage oils, formed a semicircle on one side of the bed. In the centre was a large birthing ball. Who is meant to sit on this, I wondered?

Given the vocational duty of care of midwives, it's not surprising that many of them volunteer to work overseas in conditions very different from those we are familiar with in the comforts of Australia's healthcare system. In these stories we see remarkable clinical skills and judgment in midwives – again the kind of detail rarely revealed to a lay audience. Heather Harris, in 'Sage femme', writes of an experience in Africa:

> There's no forceps here, the ventouse isn't working, exhortations to push are having little impact.
>
> '*Pousse, pousse, pousse, ma cherie!*' Time to resort to a delivery method as old as childbirth itself. Pierrette, our youngest midwife, climbs onto the narrow bed and straddles the prostrate woman . . . badgering [the uterus] to start another contraction. As the uterus wearily tightens and bulges again, Pierrette forms her

hands into fists and pushes, hard, hard, hard, on the pregnant fundus. The woman yells.

Ironically, where there is little technology, midwives are able to use their skills – usually successfully – without threats and judgment from a litigious 'client base' or peer group. As technological intervention becomes more widespread, so too does the sense of being restricted, or even undermined. This was a common theme in many of the stories.

Midwives express an often overwhelming sense of frustration – at being overworked and unable to care for mothers and children in the way their instincts want to guide them. Racing from bed to bed in busy urban hospitals, or seeing convenience and intervention overrule time-honoured methods, they occasionally express the laconic desire to work somewhere where their heart isn't so torn by all they must see and do. Two of our contributors contemplate giving up mid and working instead at a checkout in Coles or in a pie shop, but quickly admit that, despite the stress and grief, they wouldn't swap their job for any other.

Shona Davidson contrasts the feeling of being 'truly gutted' when a baby in her care dies, with the need to put on a brave face for the next patient. 'It's a cycle,' she confides, 'that goes around and around in your head, sometimes there's resolution, but more often there's not. You want to cry, you feel you should, but you're frightened to. You know that the years of accumulated grief will surge to the fore like a tidal wave and you'll drown. So, you sit there. Staring at nothing.'

It's interesting to note that while many of the writers

describe their phenomenal average daily workload, none complain that they are underpaid. They may feel undermined and undervalued, but trying to put a financial value on their work doesn't rate a mention. This is a well-recognised phenomenon in female-dominated occupations.

Many describe, instead, the bond between women and midwives, the trust that is slowly built, the sense of privilege that comes with being part of a birth experience, the triumph and exhilaration that makes any other kind of work impossible, despite the frustration. Perhaps this is because no other work could compare with the elemental nature of birth: its gruelling, awe-inspiring and intense transformation, where everything at stake is suddenly on the line. Sometimes, despite everything, babies die. Sometimes, when all seems lost, they survive. Life is fragile, and our hold on it, for all our medical wizardry and intervention, is still tenuous. The thing we are most desperate to control, resists our control. In showing us our powerlessness, though, birth also reaffirms our faith in the overwhelming human instincts of love and courage.

One disappointment in compiling this collection of stories is the absence of the male midwife voice. They are a rare group and we spoke to a few of them, but no stories were submitted. Thankfully, men – usually fathers – appear in many of the stories, but they are secondary characters – a reflection of the women-centred nature of birthing and caring for babies, a situation accepted even by men themselves.

While the quality of writing should be the driving force behind any collection of stories, it has to be remembered that most of the contributors to this book are not professional writers. The writing and editing process has been an intensive learning experience for many. (But that doesn't mean they aren't gifted in the art of storytelling, like those who write professionally.) They graphically describe the rich and diverse experiences that have shaped their working lives.

Terri Coates, a British midwife, writes that on the rare occasions when midwives appear in literature, they are 'a source of irritation rather than comfort'.[3] She exhorts midwives to write, saying: 'Midwifery and childbirth have all the ingredients required of a blockbuster novel; sex, love, anticipation, excitement, pain, exhilaration at the arrival of a new life (or the anguish of a lost baby), and the uncertainty of new relationships.' Coates' exploration of this topic provoked Jennifer Worth to write an autobiographical account of her work in the East End of London in the 1950s. Like the stories in this book, the detail is confronting, and strangely familiar.[4]

In these stories, you will hear the voices of midwives. This time, those voices won't just be comforting, encouraging, soothing, offering words of advice and support, breaking good news and tragic news, being alongside women on one of the most awe-inspiring journeys of life. They will be telling their stories, allowing you a glimpse into a world of old and new knowledge, courage, humour and, most of all, the kind of dedication that is too easy to take for granted.

As often happens when we listen properly to voices that aren't usually heard, we have been humbled by these stories, and we hope you will be too.

Notes:

1 Australian Workforce Advisory Committee, *The Midwifery Workforce in Australia, 2002–2012*, AWAC, Sydney, 2002, p. 84.

2 Amanda Tattam (ed.), *From the Heart: True stories by Australian nurses*, Lothian, Melbourne, 1997.

3 Terri Coates, 'Impressions of the midwife in literature', *Midwives Journal*, vol. 1, January 1998.

4 Jennifer Worth, *Call the Midwife*, Merton Books, Surrey, 2001.

LIFE in the LABOUR WARD

Birth in a parallel universe

LINDA FABB

I walked to work for an early shift. There had been a downpour of rain overnight after a period of unseasonal dry. The mute ambiguous tones of dawn were overwhelmed by brilliant sunshine. The world seemed to have been washed clean and fresh.

Everything had a quality of exceptional clarity. A line of water on a leaf edge cut a hot white definition between where life was nurtured and nourished, where it existed and where it did not.

My hand pushed the labour ward door open as it exploded towards me, immediately followed by an almost airborne trolley with a woman, bottom in the air, two midwives and a junior resident attached.

'Cord presentation for theatre, let them know we're on the way!' Gone.

Phone call made, I breathed in and looked up, my eyes beginning to take in the rest of the ward. What had happened overnight? Had mayhem broken loose? Every piece of equipment, usually tidily stowed away had been left, abandoned, outside the birthing rooms. Drawers hung open; leads trailed the direction of their arrival like debris washed ashore after a shipwreck in a huge storm. Both phones were ringing but seemed distant among the chaos, as if tired from being unanswered for too long. The night staff dashed from one room to the next looking focused.

Doors swishing, buzzers sounding, and the desk covered in papers and files. I noticed bloodstained water seeping out under the pan room door.

The placenta muncher had blocked again and maintenance didn't work on the weekend. I answered the phone – not one but two permanent senior staff members off sick, leaving only junior staff. They promised to send someone 'soon'. ('Soon' always scares me.) I mentioned the placenta muncher to the supervisor.

Apparently we were way over budget for maintenance, so I'm told to turn off the power and water to the unit. We are to use a muncher in one of the other labour wards until it's fixed. Great. No mention of help to clean up the mess.

As the morning staff arrived, the well-worn path of routine checking and restocking proceeded and the chaos subsided. The landscape, now more orderly, seduced us into feeling that the storm was over and we were in control.

The place was chock-a-block full and overflowing. Every bed occupied, three more women in labour on the wards and one in A&E (Accident and Emergency) waiting to be collected.

Handover at breakneck speed from strung-out night staff hyped up from running on adrenalin alone. No one had had a meal break. You could see in their faces that, despite their exhaustion, they wouldn't sleep for hours.

Room 1: Allison – Primigravida. Admitted early hours of the morning in established labour, 6 centimetres, doing well.

Room 2: Julie – Primigravida. Early labour, slow progress but appears normal.

Room 3: Mai – Multigravida. Induction for foetal growth retardation, forceps delivery with episiotomy. Awaiting transfer to the wards.

Room 4: Nicky – Primigravida. Four centimetres, requesting epidural, anaesthetist contacted.

Room 5: Alya – Multigravida. Twin pregnancy in established labour after induction yesterday. Doing well.

Room 6: Amani – Delivered but the baby was flat and sent to special care nursery. Mother extremely distressed. Speaks no English. (We can hear heartwrenching wailing from her room, like a distant survivor who has watched her baby drown.)

Room 7: Li – Multi . . .

Room 8: Caroline . . .

Prep room: Lisa . . .

My allocation – rooms 1, 2 and 3 with a student midwife.

It didn't look too bad on the face of it, but we would be busy.

Allison's face was pale with fear of a secret hidden for so long, now revealed. Small, shy and quietly spoken, she was one of the bravest women I have ever met.

She didn't say much, but what she did say was worth listening to. It was difficult to maintain eye contact with her. Over the morning her story emerged, bit by bit.

At seventeen she had been employed as a live-in nanny and was passionate about pursuing a career in this area. She had enrolled in full-time study, beginning the following year. She had become pregnant unintentionally and concealed this from her employers, who she lived with, for the entire pregnancy. She was sure she would be sacked and so much wanted to keep her job.

Yesterday morning she had gone into labour and told her employers she had the flu and returned to bed. All day she had laboured alone, waves of pain flowing through her body. Silent, not knowing how to tell them. Close the curtains, block out the world and the pains might go away. She laboured alone in the dark, the pains getting stronger, lasting longer. Consuming her now, denial banished.

In the early hours of the morning, a muffled groan had drawn her employer's attention. She had to tell her now.

'I'm pregnant,' she'd blurted. The world seemed to stop.

Her employer's face froze. Trying to conceal her shock, she asked: 'When is it due?'

'Now. I mean, it's coming. Can you call an ambulance?'

Here she is now, still alone, being very brave, trying to contain it all, process it all. What were her plans? How could I possibly meet this woman's needs on such a busy day? There isn't enough time. Obs done.

Mai and Loi were happy that their 'ordeal' was over and were both very proud of Michael, their son. He didn't need to go to the special care nursery, but a number of moderately invasive tests were to be done due to his 'low birth weight'. Neither of them were at all concerned about Michael's size. Obs done and I managed to find some food for them. Neither had eaten since yesterday morning. The ward wasn't ready for them yet. The bed wasn't empty and the ward help didn't start until 8 am. They would ring us after that.

Julie was having her first baby, had laboured all night and was getting into it. She looked frightened and tired. Husband Bruce was more interested in whether it would all be over in time for the footy and 'bringing up the boy a Magpie'.

She was doing okay. Let's hope they leave her alone.

Dr Fullofit burst into the room, pager beeping, gloved hands appearing first, followed by his mouth. The rest of him seemed to slide through the door and gradually rematerialise into a human form behind the hands.

'Time for your examination, Pauline. I hope you have progressed this time or we'll have to intervene.'

'This is Julie, Dr . . .'

'Ah, get that pager, Nurse' (never a good way to address a midwife), he said, and thrust his hip towards me. My skin crawled. Now she wouldn't be left alone.

I wished I had never thought it. I felt like I had jinxed her. I helped Julie on to the bed and instructed Bruce to hold her hand. 'Looking forward to the game, Doc? What's your team? Right-o, Nursie.'

I answered the doctor's page and headed back to the room. 'Theatre need to speak to you now,' I told him.

'Can't you see I'm up to my elbows in it?' he responded.

Message politely conveyed, I returned to find that 2 centimetres dilation in four hours wasn't satisfactory. Without a mention to Julie or Bruce, the doctor had ruptured her membranes. She lay there passive and defenceless. Nothing was said. I had a duty of care to this woman and it was now too late to mention that this was likely to increase her pain and therefore make further intervention probable, that without informed consent this action could be considered assault.

No time to discuss this privately with the doctor. Probably no point, either. All too late. Necessary obs complete, reassurance given, comfort attended. Julie's eyes begged me to stay. Mai's bed was ready and A&E was hassling.

I don't have enough time.

Paperwork checked. Labels checked and rechecked. Transfer complete. Didn't really get time to say goodbye. Down to A&E to collect Basra. Use the stairs – it's quicker.

Basra was Somalian and had received no antenatal care. Her husband had forbidden it, as the hospital was unable to guarantee all-female care. She was 22, and spoke fluent Somali, French and German. I only speak English. We would need an interpreter. She had been circumcised as a child, and the scar would now need to be cut open before birth. I wasn't looking forward to that. Settled in, obs done, doctor called and interpreter paged.

Back to Julie half an hour later and her contractions had increased dramatically. Pethidine was called for and, shortly after, an epidural requested. The cascade of intervention had been started and was taking off, full steam ahead.

Into room 5 now to do a set of obs for my colleague. Ayla was in labour with twins. She already had two children. She was being induced 'before they got too big' and was wired for sound. Monitor leads and drips hung from her like seaweed, limiting her movement, threatening to drown her. She was experiencing severe back pain with contractions as she sat in her bed – marooned.

If only I could get her up and into a better position. Buzzer ringing frantically in room 4. Must go. Need more time.

Nicky and Steve were having their first baby. They were also both intravenous heroin users. Nicky had been labouring all night and had been requesting an epidural for four hours now. They both looked strung out. I told them that I would page the anaesthetist again but believed he was in theatre. Steve was getting anxious and pacing around the room, kicking the walls as he reached them.

'As if that will do any bloody good,' he replied, having heard this too many times already. I paged the anaesthetist; he was in theatre, but the message was to be conveyed. 'Junkies' are always put to the bottom of the list, as if their pain isn't real, or they should be punished for their addiction. This always seemed like such a self-defeating approach.

Back to Julie. She's not coping so well now. Bruce has gone off for a fag and is nowhere to be found. It would be great if he was here to help her walk around.

Need more tim . . .

Back to Allison. Her world has shrunk and her focus is inward. Her time is drawing closer. The student midwife seems like an angel, sitting with her, holding her hand. I'm so grateful someone is there for her. She almost looks as scared as Allison did. This isn't fair. More ti . . .

More obs, more buzzers and phones answered, more paging, more running – more, more, more. No time to talk, no time to really use my skills, no time to do my job properly.

The anaesthetist arrived to insert Julie's epidural. Procedure completed, the foetal heart rate dropped and she was off to theatre in twenty minutes. I reminded him about Nicky and asked if he could make it a priority as her husband was getting very agitated.

Back to Basra. Still no interpreter. I try the telephone interpreter service. I wait for ten minutes just to talk to someone. They are ringing around Australia trying to find someone. Page the doctor again.

Allison's expression was intense as I walked in. She looked directly into my eyes.

'I want the baby adopted out.'

It took me a minute to catch my breath. Had she thought about this? Does she understand the process? What are her wishes regarding contact with her baby after birth? No time now to discuss this. No time. Three buzzes from room 4. The universal signal for COME NOW.

As I enter the room I find a student midwife pinned to the bed by the throat with one of Steve's hands; the other, in a fist, is heading towards me.

'Stay cool,' I think. I can understand his anger. I manage to swing the monitor between us and he misses. He is really losing the plot now. More staff arrive, security is called and Steve is removed. Nicky still didn't get her epidural. There is talk of assault charges. No one mentions charging the anaesthetist with neglect. In the middle of all this I'm called out of the room for a phone call.

It's a close friend of mine. 'Hello, Linda. It's Hunter.' His voice is quiet and soothing. 'I just wanted to let you know that we had a beautiful baby girl, Ellya, this morning at home . . . It was magical. A wonderful and amazing experience to watch Robyn safe in our home, birthing our baby with such calm confidence, and knowing power . . . They are both really well. They are breastfeeding as we speak . . . The midwives were fantastic. They were with us during the whole labour. No drugs, no stitches, all very straightforward. It's all very calm and happy here . . . We have saved the placenta and would like you to come and plant a cherry tree on it with us one day . . . How's your day going?'

His voice wraps around me like a warm blanket, comforting and nurturing me. I take a deep breath and absorb the calm and everydayness of it. There *is* another way . . . It doesn't need to be like this . . . The chaos has dissolved around me and I feel joy for the first time that day.

Allison birthed her baby boy with courage and bravery. She named him Cameron and kept him in hospital with her for a week and breastfed him. She wanted to give him the best start she could. The social workers were horrified, but the midwives supported her all the way. Then she adopted him out. She felt she had very little to offer her boy at this time in her life and was emotionally ill-equipped to be a single mother. She believed he would have a much better chance in the world with adoptive parents and hoped she would be able to maintain contact. I often wonder what happened to her.

Mai and Loi's baby Michael was found to be normal and healthy despite being small. His older siblings were recorded to be a similar weight at birth. Mai was only 138 centimetres in height and weighed 48 kilograms. Loi was of similar build. Discharge conclusion: 'Probably of normal weight for this family background!'

Julie and Bruce's baby girl was born by Caesarean section and both did well until Julie developed a severe wound infection leading to her being unable to breastfeed. Bruce thought this was best anyway.

Basra was still in labour when I left work. Thoughts of the horror of what she had to go through prevented me from following her up.

The twins were also born by Caesarean section and were in the intensive care nursery with respiratory difficulties.

I was always too scared to find out what became of Nicky and Steve. I wonder if the system supported them in parenthood, or if it just reinforced their demise?

Amani spoke no English and an interpreter hadn't been available. Her sister-in-law had been used to interpret, as this was the only option available. She had misunderstood some of what was said and told Amani the baby was being taken away to die. The baby was actually fine. Mother and baby were happily reunited, immediately after an interpreter was found at 12.30 pm. Her painful wails can now be understood.

We did plant a cherry tree over Ellya's placenta, and every summer we enjoy handfuls of the best cherries I have ever tasted.

Full circle

SHANNON MORRIS

I will never forget the first slip of wet black hair that I watched emerge from between a mother's legs. I will never cease to think that a pregnant belly is beautiful or lactating breasts amazing. I will never forget how magical women's bodies are and how strong woman can be if we allow them. This is my journey from student to midwife.

Thursday, 7 March

One of the women I am caring for today is in tears. It's her first day as a mother. When I meet her she is staring at the wall and crying, her breast uncovered, her baby lying across her lap. She looks up at me and says, 'I didn't think it would be this hard.'

I listen to her cry; I acknowledge that it's hard work. She comforts her baby for a while, holds him, loves him. He nuzzles into her neck and she can feel his warm breath and soft hair.

I get her to take a deep breath, drop her shoulders and blow out all her tension. Then we talk for a bit about how she thought it would be, how it really is, and how things will change and become different, and challenging, and easier. I tell her again that both she and her baby are on a steep learning curve, they are in a whole new world – but at least they are together and they can learn.

Wednesday, 13 March

Today I was the receiver of baby girl, Sophia Rose, born by elective Caesarean section. Just seconds old, mother under general anaesthetic, and I was left holding the baby.

I saw hundreds of Caesareans when I was an anaesthetic nurse, but then I knew nothing of the woman or her family other than what I could scrounge from notes and theatre room chatter.

This mum had an emergency Caesarean with her first daughter when good, strong contractions produced no baby. She had a general anaesthetic then, and wanted one this time, too.

In the morning I'd helped her get ready for theatre, put in a catheter, done the clip, checked out her old scar, felt her baby move and listened to its heartbeat. We talked about breastfeeding. I met her husband, her mother and her father, was shown pictures of her daughter, and talked to her sister on the phone. We talked about names for this baby; we all got excited as the time drew near.

I was nervous and excited about receiving this baby. It was like I was going to meet an old friend. Sophia was born at 12.44 pm. She was pink and screaming. I put my hand on her chest and could feel her heart beating. I could feel her umbilical cord still pulsing even though it had been cut from her mother. I dried her off, clamped and cut her cord a little shorter, wrapped her up warmly and took her out to meet her dad.

Friday, 15 March

Just before 2.30 pm an amazingly calm, strong woman came in with her husband. We did a quick abdominal palpation and listened for a foetal heart. She jumped up for another contraction and said she had a lot of pressure – membranes ruptured, contraction over, off to the loo.

She said she really wanted to get down on her knees, so we put a mat and sheet on the floor and bolstered up the end with a beanbag and some pillows. She put on a very pretty nightie and shed her knickers. Down on her knees, she wanted to push. As she did, her perineum bulged outwards. Next push, head on view, peri stretched beautifully; I could see her baby's brow. And then . . . pop! A face, eyes open and looking around. We put a mirror down so that she could see, too. We waited for the next contraction, and her baby simply slid out. She went straight into her mother's arms all slippery and wet. And there was this lovely family and a wonderfully alert baby, all looking at each other.

Her GP, who missed the whole thing, popped in to see how she was. There was a bit of discussion about what time her baby was born. The doctor said that in 21 years he had never looked to see what time it was when a baby was born. The conversation that followed was this:

Mum: 'Wow, in 21 years you must have delivered a lot of babies.'

Doctor: 'No, I haven't delivered any, but I've seen a lot of mothers deliver theirs.'

I liked him instantly. A lot.

Sunday, 14 April

My first birth. Well, sort of – my hands *were* on the bottom of the rest.

Maryanne arrived at about 6 am and had been having fairly regular contractions through the night, so not much sleep. This was her second baby. She had laboured well for her first, but seemed to get stuck somewhere in the dilation process and the birth ended as a Caesarean. She was very keen to have this baby vaginally, and I was keen to help her.

She breathed and laughed early in the day. When things got tougher we walked, used heat packs, tried a bath, and used different positions and lots of coaching to focus on slowing the panic breathing. Then her GP turned up.

He wanted to know what was going on in there. He wanted to augment her labour in some way, so he ruptured the membranes. He started talking about pain-relief options – he thought it was too early for nitrous oxide, so there was pethidine or an epidural.

She opted for an epidural at 8 centimetres dilation. Baby wasn't born for another five hours and now we had continuous CTG monitoring! Can't help thinking that without it labour wouldn't have lasted as long. But she was comfortable and the baby was fine.

For the birth of the baby's head my hand had sort of hovered – not really sure what it was supposed to be doing but with plenty of instructions being hurled from midwife and doctor – God knows what poor Maryanne thought.

The baby started to turn to face me, but the doctor decided she might want to go the other way! Luckily she just kept coming, but not before another set of hands came out of the blue to get in on the action, pulling and shoving. This baby wasn't so much born as yanked from her mother's body. All blue and floppy, I guided her up to her mother's breast. The placenta was born. Maryanne had a bit of a tear – was that us? They assure me not.

It was special to feel a newborn slide through my hands, so why then did I get in my car at the end of the day and cry? I was completely overwhelmed. Birth wasn't at all the way I thought it would be. She had had a vaginal birth after a Caesarean, she had a daughter, she was breastfeeding, and she was ecstatic. I was ecstatic for her for all of those things, but as a midwife-to-be, did I have it all wrong? Why do we say we 'catch' a baby as it's born, if I'd just been shown to pull?

Monday, 22 April

What an absolute buzz. I caught a baby all on my own. He slipped into my hands and I brought him up to meet his mum, who could hardly believe what had just happened.

There was no pulling or pushing. I talked to her as his head crowned, waited for him to restitute and then caught him on the way out.

She laboured beautifully: so internally focused, so in tune with her body and, it seemed, also in tune with my voice and that of her mother. If she began to cry out during a contraction or to hyperventilate, all I had to say was ‘breathe’ or ‘slow’, and instantly she was back in focus and on top of the contraction again. She used heat, water and focus, breathing and positional changes, but no drugs; she never asked, we never offered.

Tuesday, 23 April

Afternoons are good to me. I met one of the GPs coming up the stairs at the start of the shift. He was on his way to see Ann, a lovely woman with an ‘irritable’ uterus. Ann was 38-and-a-bit weeks pregnant and extremely uncomfortable with groin pain, and had been having irregular contractions for a couple of days. She also had four boys at home and was getting pretty sick of the whole thing. To make a long story a bit shorter, her GP broke her membranes and we sat and waited for something to happen.

It took quite a few hours for the contractions to take on a regular feel, though they became stronger very rapidly. Her previous labours had all been quite quick – the last less than two hours – so there was a lot of frustration about why this one was so different. We talked between contractions; saying that this one was an induction, the babe was a bit posterior, and that it was its own little person and would come out its own way. The three of us – her husband was there, too – worked through letting the other labours go and just concentrating on this one. She walked, ate, drank, used the birth ball, and just sat and breathed, too.

I guess at about 7 pm the contractions changed, gaining both momentum and strength. It was nothing anyone said, just the look of her; the talking stopped and concentration replaced the concern on her face. I got her some hot packs, and my gut told me to move her to one of the birthing rooms.

I got her comfy on the mat, leaning over a chair. Saying 'call me if you need me', I ducked out to quickly update my notes when I heard that growl of a noise that I know would rapidly be a push. I raced back inside and barely had time to get her knickers off and my gloves on and there he was. I'm quite proud of myself; it was a very nice catch! I passed him through her legs and ducked around the front to read her reaction: disappointed, maybe, momentarily. 'Oh, it's a boy. I could've sworn he was a girl.'

Monday, 13 May

Preadmissions booking clinic – it's quite draining. I didn't realise how lucky I am until I started listening to other people's lives. Stillbirths, terminations for various reasons (among them Down's syndrome), multiple miscarriages, marriages falling apart after planning a child, drug addiction, finding yourself pregnant and away from family and friends, or just not having any family or friends.

I'm constantly amazed at how honest people are, how trusting they are with the information of their lives. I mean, it's private stuff. I'm a complete stranger asking really intimate questions. Maybe it's the first time anyone has really asked, or listened to the answer.

Confidentiality is everywhere in healthcare, but it's never been so in-my-face before. Not in such a big way. This stuff is about sex and families and life, it's fascinating and raw – and so are the emotions.

Monday, 10 June

Saw an episiotomy today. I'm not really sure what was going on, there was no distress for either mum or babe, but the woman had the most swollen peri/labia/genitals I have ever seen. I think that the baby would have come out through there; it was very stretchy despite the swelling. Maybe she would have torn, and I have honestly no idea to what degree. But the consensus between midwife and doctor is that it would have been very bad.

She had an epidural – which had pretty much worn off – in some kind of 'deal' that I'm not so sure was made with her. The syringe had run out and just never got refilled – better for pushing, 'they said'. And her peri was so swollen there wasn't anywhere to put a local, so she had to try desperately to suck in enough gas to dull the pain while she was sewn back together.

Overall, I feel sick.

Friday, 14 June

I thought today would be a lovely day to see a baby born. The woman is Indian and quietly and confidently rocking her way through labour with her own breath and focus. She is tired, having already been in this place for twenty hours or so, but everything looks good.

At some point it doesn't anymore. First, there is Synto (Syntocinon) added at 7 centimetres or so, and then there is mec (meconium). Then she is fully dilated and, despite her best efforts, the babe won't budge. We are fooled for a little while, but it doesn't actually 'progress'. Then there is deceleration in foetal heart rate, variable and not long after, late. The mec is thick, the babe is distressed, the poor woman is on her back, legs in stirrups, forceps gleaming on the table.

Another midwife comes into the room and demands to know why we have moved the bed. Very early on, I had moved it to the edge of the room, out of the way, so that she had maximum space to wander and just be. The light had been low, the curtains drawn. The room is now lit up like Christmas, but not nearly so pretty.

She is given a pudendal block, and the doctor looks at me while she hacks an episiotomy, commenting on how effective her block is: 'Look at her face; she's very relaxed and has no idea what I'm doing.' The episiotomy is extended three times before the baby is born.

I am shaking violently while I try to suck the thick mec from his mouth, and then he is out and gone to the resuscitation trolley in the blink of an eye. A tiny baby, covered in green slime.

I look around at his mother, who seems completely unaware of anything, at his father who is pale and clammy, torn between his wife and newborn son, and his grandmother standing like a statue in the far corner of the room.

There is commotion over by the crib, but I can hear a lusty cry. Third stage is some kind of blur, and the repair is started the instant the placenta is out because the bleeding from her wound is quite profuse.

I am aware that I'm doing things to try and assist this woman, turning up the drip to try and control the bleeding, talking to her, fetching suture material, but I become nauseated and have to leave the room. I feel that I have let her down, not because of the type of birth, but because I could offer her nothing. Outside I shake and quietly cry; I think I am in shock.

I know that baby was in trouble and I know he needed to get out, but it was like a scene from *The Texas Chainsaw Massacre* in there. I rang my husband and told him I couldn't do it anymore, it's not what I thought it would be, I'm no good at it and I just can't do this job. I don't want to feel like vomiting when a baby is born, and I don't want to cry because I'm so distressed – I want to cry because it's wonderful.

Saturday, 22 June

Really busy day. No catches, but a baby born.

His birth was an emergency Caesarean. It was pretty horrible. Apparently earlier in the day, after numerous poor-looking CTGs, lots of tears and no dilation, she had asked for a Caesarean and was told that everything would be okay and it was best for the baby to be born vaginally.

So there she was, at half past two in the afternoon, flat on her back in stirrups with some kind of PVC cone thing shoved up her vagina while a doctor took several attempts at a foetal scalp pH. It went from bad to worse, and twenty minutes later she was in theatre under general anaesthetic because she was such an emotional wreck she couldn't distinguish pressure from pain.

Her husband was in the corridor sobbing uncontrollably – a tower of a man reduced to rubble on my shoulder, so much so that I stayed with him while another midwife went in to receive their baby – who was fine. When given the all clear I went in and got his son from the theatre and brought him out to his dad, which set off another round of tears and a new fear that his wife wouldn't be okay. She was fine, too.

Birth is scary stuff.

Sunday, 28 July

There is a reason a girl needs five sisters: to be surrounded by strength and love in labour.

Today's was a beautiful birth, a beautiful family.

Amanda wasn't far away from giving birth to her second son when I met her. She was doing a great job of leaning over the bed and breathing long and hard through the peak of the pains. Her sisters and mother and husband were all there, rubbing her back and giving encouragement every step of the way. It was quite a sight and I felt very superfluous – but in a good way.

Every now and then I listened to the baby, and when Amanda's noises changed to odd grunts I watched her more closely. She fluffed around looking for her husband's old T-shirt, which she wanted to be wearing when she gave birth. And after a few more odd little grunts and with the T-shirt in place, I asked if I could have a quick peek, to see if I could see anything like a baby's head.

I ended up doing birth by mirror. Amanda wanted to see, and because she was squatting quite low to the ground, with her husband on one side and a sister on the other, it was an easy solution to give her a better view.

With a reasonable bit of head on view, something was holding the babe back. I asked Amanda what she needed from me.

I knew her first babe had been born from a standing position. With one push (and only one) he had hit the floor, and she had had a nasty third-degree tear. I now imagined she was experiencing quite a bit of terror about her new babe's wellbeing.

I told her that she was in a perfect position to catch her own baby. Quick as a flash she said she didn't want to, but pleaded with me to make sure I did. I promised her I would catch her baby and not let it fall, and I told her to go with her body and ease her little person out gently.

She pushed beautifully, following her body's lead. Very gently his little face swept her perineum and then he tumbled out into my hands. Amanda wept with joy and that wonderful birth room stacked with family came alive to the sound of his cry.

I am so lucky to meet such strong women, families and tiny souls.

Monday, 5 August

Why is it that when you learn about breastfeeding it's on pert little breasts with tiny round nipples that poke out, and with a baby that has a big hungry mouth that just wants to feed?

It's just not like that, is it? What about the large breasts with nipples that are underneath and flat? And why do those mothers always seem to have babies with the tiniest mouth you have ever seen, and who just aren't interested even though they are starving?

Thursday, 5 September

I quite like to watch other midwives 'do' birth. Some love to panic, some need to do stuff, others do nothing. Some rush in and cut the cord as a matter of immediate priority, and others only remember to cut it when the baby can't go to Dad for a cuddle because the cord isn't long enough.

Why do some of us do it one way and others another? What little bits of our brains make us comfortable or not? I can feel my way emerging.

Saturday, 7 September

Looked up my own birth in the birth register tonight. How weird was that? I was 4040 grams, born at 12.34 pm, and caught by pupil midwife Stanhope while Dr Jolley looked on. It was the strangest feeling to see me written down like that – it made me feel almost famous.

Monday, 16 September

Today I feel like a midwife. Today I'm so sure that I'm doing the right thing and that I love it. Today I didn't catch a baby, but instead talked a dad through it – it was magic. Telling you makes me grin.

When I told the other students at dinner, they said I must have heaps of births if I'm giving them away – but I didn't give it to anyone. It's not mine to give.

Her story for you. Her fourth baby (sixth pregnancy), his first. Her eighteen-year-old daughter was there; she wasn't happy about the pregnancy and had no plans to be there for the birth. But her mother's membranes ruptured – labour established – and she was stuck.

It was nice just to let her mother do her own thing. She found a comfy spot and she laboured. I tidied the space, listened to the foetal heart, offered encouragement and comfort to all. I asked who was catching the baby. The dad said he worked on a farm and had caught pigs and lambs and calves, and I agreed that they were all slippery little things. So, when the time came, I told him he'd better come behind her. Her daughter then held her mum's hand.

The baby's head birthed and, while he waited for her body to emerge, the dad massaged her tiny head. I told him which way she would turn, and a beautiful baby girl was born gently into her daddy's big hands while the other midwife and I watched.

We passed her through her mother's legs, skin to skin, and the four members of the family cried, all hugging each other.

I think it's good for children to see their siblings born, even if they didn't mean to.

Thursday, 11 December

I have been motivated to start writing birth stories again because today I watched another father catch his child. What made it so special was that the woman was Lucy, and the birth of her daughter some 21 months ago was the very first birth I witnessed as a baby midwife.

I scrolled back through this journal to find my story of that birth, and it's amazing how similar they are. Same beautiful strong woman, the same quiet, internalised pain, same pretty cotton nightie, same nice doctor.

Lucy got to the hospital at about 9.45 am. After very quick hellos and 'I remember you', she ducked into the loo. I grabbed a mat and a beanbag, because she said she'd like to birth on the floor. I then talked to her husband about when things had really started and how their other children were.

Lucy was beautiful, still smiling. When she put on her nightie, I instantly recognised it as the same one she had birthed in last time. Then she just knelt down on the mat and laboured. I felt one contraction and, just as I did, I felt her membranes 'pop' through her abdomen. We waited for the contraction to end, then I helped her with her knickers and called out that a warm bundle and a phone call to her doctor would be a good idea. It was 10.05 am.

Her husband asked me if this was 'it', if it was all happening. I said I was pretty sure it was, and asked if he'd like to catch his baby. He came around behind her and with the next contraction his son's head advanced slowly and calmly into his waiting hands. His little head turned and then, with my hands just alongside, we slipped him shoulder by shoulder out of his mother and to his daddy.

He rested him gently between Lucy's knees, and when she had recovered from the effort of his birth she looked down and picked him up and brought him to her chest. A perfect son at 10.11 am.

The doctor arrived just after his birth and I heard his smile through the curtain, if that is possible, when he heard their son cry.

Birthing is so special. Today I felt like a midwife and I remembered why I love my job so much – not so much for what I did, because I'm not actually sure that I 'did' anything, so perhaps more for what I didn't do.

Lucy's baby breastfed just as simply and naturally as his sister did before him. And Lucy and her husband basked in the glory of greeting their newborn without intrusion or procedures. It was great to be a part of that again. Welcome to the world, little one.

Three hundred midwives at the drop of a hat

NOLA AICKEN

For some years now there has been much unrest in our regional maternity unit.

The main problems seem to be insufficient funds for an already crippled healthcare system and the pervasiveness of the obstetrical model of care. The cutbacks are constant, and interventions in childbirth are commonplace and accepted as everyday procedures.

When I wrote this story in late 2002, the midwives in our unit were rebelling. We were faced with not only the reduction to our women/staffing ratio, but the possible closure of some of our birth suites. At the time, we had seven birth rooms (three of which were double bed suites where the couple could remain following the birth) and an assessment room. We boasted

1200 births a year, and were concerned for the safety of the women and babies in our care – we wanted only the best for them.

The blood sample seemed to freeze in time . . . as it dropped from my hand in slow motion into the waiting esky. Suddenly I was hit by the chaos around me.

After a quiet day at the community midwives clinic, I had travelled back to the hospital at 2 pm, instead of the usual 4 pm close. The unit was overflowing. The postnatal rooms were full. The birth rooms were full. The midwife in charge, at the end of her tether, was fractious and snapping. There was the clinical manager, near tears. Staff flew about in all directions.

A woman, obviously having contractions, stood in the entrance foyer. Her husband was beside her. A midwife came rushing over. 'Nola, can you possibly assess this woman who has just arrived and is most likely in labour?' she asked. She hastily added that the woman thought she had spontaneous rupture of membranes.

'I don't mind in the least.' I was there to help until my home time, anyway. I could see that the woman wasn't going to be assessed for quite a while. Not only did they not have a room available, but they had no available midwives. As it was, the clinical manager had been ringing around for the past two hours trying to find a midwife who could work.

It was an interesting situation, particularly in the light of our director of nursing's recent appearance on the television news. In response to reports of escalating industrial tension in the maternity unit, she claimed there was no real problem. 'There are 300 midwives who can be called at the drop of a hat!' she had stated.

We had been fighting management's plans for months. They wanted to close labour rooms and reduce staff in Maternity. We believed that the rooms had to stay open because we use them constantly, and that women's safety is affected if we don't have adequate staff ratios.

I introduced myself to the couple now sitting in the foyer. 'Laura and Bruce, my name is Nola. Would you like to come with me to the women's health clinic?'

It was 2.30 pm when I settled Laura into the assessment room and attached the CTG straps. Laura was uncomfortable with her contractions. 'Can I stand up?' she asked.

'Yes, Laura. As soon as I have this machine connected and going, I'll give you a hand to get up.'

I was finishing her observations, when she gasped. There was fluid running down her legs. I checked her pad, which showed a meconium-stained colour that we midwives don't like to see. Laura's membranes had ruptured at home at 1 pm and the leaking had continued. I needed to advise the midwife in charge and the resident doctor. Laura was obviously going nowhere, now that meconium-stained liquor was evident.

Laura's contractions were regular but mild. She had a birth plan which requested no interventions: midwife care, active labour; Bruce to cut the cord; the baby to stay with Laura; no Syntocinon for Laura (physiological third stage); no Konakion, Vitamin K or Hepatitis B injections for the baby.

The meconium-stained liquor had changed the situation somewhat, because now we not only had to closely observe the baby via a monitor but we had to have a medical person at the birth to aspirate airways. Early cutting of the cord could also be very likely.

We worked through the expected scenarios together, and I reassured Laura that some of their plans could still go ahead, as long as her labour was straightforward.

I left the room soon after to collect the tympanic and returned to find Laura kneeling on the floor vomiting into a towel I had provided earlier. *Hmmmm.* She was moving along with this labour and it was time to find a birth room quickly.

The only room vacant was a double bed suite. Usually women with meconium-stained liquor are placed in the single rooms because of the need to observe them closely, but all the singles were full.

Once settled in the room, Laura asked to kneel on the floor. I set up a mattress for her and brought in the equipment we needed, including the women's health CTG as it was the only monitor available.

I was pleased that Laura was now comfortable and could get on with her labour. She was an internal labourer and went into herself with the contractions with a bare murmur, but I could see that her contractions were hotting up. They were lasting longer and she was concentrating more with them. I caught up on my notes and set up the birth trolley. I had a feeling that Laura was on a roll.

Given the rapidly moving situation, I hadn't yet examined her to confirm the position of the baby. I explained to Laura that when she was ready, she could lie on the mattress while I carried out a quick palpation. Babe's head was well in the pelvis, so I relaxed and felt we were ready now for the pending birth. At 3 pm Laura again vomited, but was otherwise in good control. She was using a wheat pack, and Bruce pressed her lower back firmly as she kneeled forward against the side of the bed to manage the contractions.

The politics outside were interesting. Where were the 300 midwives today? The midwife in charge had asked if I was prepared to work a double shift and suggested that I request triple time for my efforts. (A nurse in the emergency department had been given triple time recently, when they were unable to find any available staff.)

In normal circumstances I would have been happy to work, just for Laura's sake. But with our recent industrial dispute and the fact that the hospital board appeared to have little interest in the safety of our women, I only agreed to work if I was given triple time. The clinical manager's quick response was that I could finish after all at 4.30 pm, as she was sure that one of the women labouring in the other rooms would have had their baby by that time. The poor midwife working with that woman could then take over my room, write up the previous birth, carry out postnatal care for the other woman and her baby, move her to the postnatal area and also manage Laura. When midwives are run ragged, it's no wonder we feel stressed.

Just after 3 pm the clinical manager caught up with me again and offered me double time if I was prepared to work a double shift. I accepted and got on with the job at hand.

Returning to Laura's room with a heat pack, I arrived just as the resident doctor, with a medical student in tow, was about to enter following a brief knock. While I was expecting them to visit due to Laura's meconium stained liquor, I had hoped they would knock and then wait at the door for permission to enter.

Attempting to slow the doctor up, I called out: 'Are you okay?'

'Just wanting to see what's going on here!' the doctor said as she continued to bustle inside.

This doctor had spent some time with us before as an obstetric/gynaecology resident and had proved to be super-enthusiastic and promising, but she didn't seem to have much idea about a labouring woman's need for privacy as she birthed. She was always in a rush, always wanting to do examinations in the whisk of a moment. She had often ruffled my feathers with her inability to recognise what labouring women need. More often than not, I attempted to get around her with quiet determination, rather than war zone tactics, because, despite her manner, she did have a genuine interest in the wellbeing of the women in her care.

Standing over Laura, the doctor loudly introduced herself and her enthusiastic follower, who was already making me feel irritable, as he moved about in a very medical manner observing the CTG and Laura's notes. The doctor continued to question Laura, while I continued to ask her not to do so while Laura was having contractions and attempting to focus with her labour.

The doctor went on regardless, asking to carry out an abdominal palpation. I again felt irritated by the lack of recognition of my own notes or palpation. When Laura was ready she did lie back on the mattress, despite finding this difficult as her contractions were now doubling and she had little rest between – I felt she was demonstrating late first stage. The doctor presumed that

Laura wouldn't mind if the medical student also examined her. Steam was coming out of my ears as Laura tried to face the next contraction on her back.

Obviously in some discomfort, she made a half-hearted attempt to return to her previous position as hands continued to explore her abdomen. I moved forward and, pushing the student's hands aside, helped Laura up with Bruce's help. They hadn't finished, though. The doctor again stood over Laura and asked to carry out a vaginal examination.

'Laura's obstetrician will want an examination done,' she said.

To my horror, the medical student also appeared to be expecting a repeat opportunity for practice, rolling up his sleeves and scanning the room for gloves, hoping that he could also do a vaginal exam. Nipping his plans in the bud, I told the doctor that I expected her to be quick about it. This was no time for a student to take an opportunity at Laura's expense, particularly when she was having little reprieve between contractions.

Fortunately the doctor was quick, and we had Laura back in her position as the next contraction assaulted her body. It was now 3.25 pm. The doctor announced that Laura was 4 centimetres dilated, some shortening of the cervix was yet to occur and the head wasn't down far enough.

I smiled to myself at that conclusion! Interesting, when Laura's body language was demonstrating something completely different. However, the doctor seemed happy now. With a quick suggestion to the student that he may like to remain in the room and observe Laura's progress, she was gone in a flash.

Noooo! This was all we needed. A young man standing around and staring at a labouring woman! I had already reassured Laura that 4 centimetres meant nothing at all. One minute, multigravidas can be 4 centimetres, and the next fully dilated.

Laura asked to go to the toilet, so I unplugged the machinery and helped her into the bathroom, thinking that a few moments of privacy may be beneficial for her. I asked the student if he might like to go and make himself a coffee. I said that Laura was an internal labourer and so he might not see much action for a while. He was relieved, and left enthusiastically.

Now, I felt, we could get back to the focus of labour without disruption. Suddenly we heard Laura calling Bruce into the bathroom, and as we rushed in, she was standing over the toilet with undies around her hips, appearing distressed. She was feeling loads of pressure. I had a quick look and could see nothing, but taking note of the sound in her voice, I quickly helped her over to the bed. Dropping over the beanbag, she then made a noise indicating surprise – or was it pain?

'I feel like pushing!' she gasped.

Pants down! Head on view! Yeeessss! Emergency buzzer on! Gloves! No need for anything else. Then the cavalry arrived – charging through the door with the doctor in the lead, as if on the heels of the retreating enemy. The resuscitation trolley was banged and bashed through the door.

'Do you have the suction ready?' the doctor called out loudly.

'Yes, it's ready.'

A midwife called out, 'Do you have Syntocinon?'

'No – don't need it. Physiological third stage!' I replied.

The medical student was in my face. So much for that private moment of birth! While I concentrated on reassuring Laura and observing the wonderful arrival of this little baby, there seemed to be pandemonium around us. Had there not been meconium we wouldn't have needed the rabblerousers, so I tried to ignore them all.

Laura was gently pushing her baby out and I talked to her as she progressed. She was doing beautifully. At 3.45 pm her little babe was born and I caught him nicely. I couldn't help but smile as the student tried to assist me – if he only knew how many babies I have caught over the years!

The doctor had aspirated the little fellow's airways on the perineum and now she offered the scissors to Bruce. My estimation of her suddenly rose a notch. She was clearly keen for the baby to be transferred to the resuscitation cot for further aspiration, but she allowed Bruce to cut the cord before the babe was whisked away. We had a brief reprieve as the attention in the room was focused on the baby.

Laura moved awkwardly over on to her back and leaned against the beanbag to deliver the placenta. I suggested she may like to squat and as she did, the doctor and the student suddenly realised that this third stage was a little different from the usual.

I hadn't made a fuss about Laura's request for physiological third stage, as I have found in the past that the less said, the better for the mother. Some midwives and doctors are nervous about the idea, as an 'active' third stage is a more common practice in our large obstetric unit.

Years of attending homebirths have taught me to be very comfortable with the normal process of physiological third stage, which occurs without the administering of an oxytocic and controlled cord traction. The doctor and the student were now observing at close hand what was happening with the placenta.

Laura squatted and then said, 'Here it comes.' The placenta passed easily into my hands and into the dish. So, with a quick check of Laura's perineum (which was intact) and the fundus (firm and central), the doctor and her assistant departed – the cavalry was gone!

Following the clamping of the cord and weighing the baby (2980 grams), I then snuggled the little fellow – still naked – into his mother's breast.

The endless cleaning up and writing up of notes awaited me, and so I left the little family alone to enjoy their baby in privacy. Oscar Jack was now in his mother's arms with a proud father close by. Apart from the few interruptions endured with much tolerance by Laura and Bruce, this was a great day and a great birth.

The industrial action begun in late 2002 finally ended in early 2003. The outcomes for our maternity unit were mainly positive. For the time being all birth rooms would remain open, other than the closure of one small suite which was to become the lactation consultant's office. The midwives were reassured that staff cutbacks wouldn't occur without adequate consultation with all maternity staff. At the time of writing, there has been no final decision on the women/staffing ratio.

Fathers make great catchers

LARAINE HOOD

Why is it that when some men make the transition to fatherhood, and have been present at a birth, they automatically assume the title of honorary midwife? I have seen this happen so often, usually with hilarious results. Having survived the embarrassment of becoming a tad unstuck, the men usually realise that midwives do actually have some knowledge and expertise, after all.

One such incident occurred during a beautiful water birth. This particular father had been present at a previous water birth and so, in addition to his role as honorary midwife, he assumed the position of water-birth expert as well. His long-suffering wife was contracting beautifully, encompassed in a fog of warm water and endorphins that strongly and surely supported her in the journey towards the imminent birth.

At one stage, I had a brief conversation with the woman, between contractions and sips of juice. We discussed her progress and agreed that we didn't need to do a vaginal examination.

The budding honorary midwife agreed, and said that when he last checked the cervix it was about 7 centimetres dilated because he could fit three fingertips between the circular edges! At first I thought he was joking, but I soon realised he was serious when he held up his size 9 hand to verify the measurement.

His wife, leaning back against him in the water, seemed blissfully unaware of our discussion and had tuned out to relax before the next contraction came.

Labour progressed beautifully. After a brief episode of transition, when she told him to leave the birth tub and he began to tell her she didn't mean it because she was transitional, thankfully the urge to push overwhelmed her. He, of course, was 'coaching', but she was tuned into her body, only pushing when the urge overcame her, not when the increasingly frustrated coach instructed.

Just as the baby's head crowned, he moved around so as to be able to catch the baby. The three of us had already discussed her wish to birth this baby into her own hands. When I gently reminded him of her wishes, he barked back at me that this was *his* baby, not mine, and *he* would catch it. I gave him the benefit of the doubt and assumed he was 'transitional' himself, and not just being chauvinistically rude.

The woman kept breathing her baby out, very calm and focused. The baby had emerged to the neck, when suddenly the father put his hands on the head as if to pull.

'Don't pull!' I told him quickly. 'Just let her gently push the baby out at her own pace.'

Again, he gave me a look that told me I was a complete idiot and unless I wanted to be drowned forthwith, I should shut up as he was the one directing proceedings. While I was considering this, he calmly announced: 'I've got the cord now, the baby will be out soon,' and proceeded to pull something towards him.

At this point, my blood froze. To pull the cord in this manner would be a disaster.

The mother let out the most primal of screams and pushed with unbelievable maternal courage. Driven by adrenalin and that scream, I immediately sprang into action to prevent what I perceived as impending disaster.

Then suddenly I saw the most triumphant look on her face. She brought her baby daughter to the surface in her hands, tears of joy running down her face. The baby opened her eyes, gave a small whimper and was immediately clasped tightly to her mother's chest – an absolute triumph of birth and womanhood. There were tears all around as this beautiful baby girl easily took her first breaths and met her family.

The father? Oh, yes, instead of a loop of cord, he had a handful of poo. Fortunately, we were all so attentive to the new baby girl, he was able to discard his 'cord' quietly, which slightly reduced his embarrassment. I did manage to catch his eye, though, and give him a rather mischievous wink.

I'm glad that nothing was said at the time, but it's one of those images stored in my midwife's brain to smile about, on days when life is a bit rainy and I need a ray of sunshine.

A tale of two fruits

JOANNE VINE

At some stage in her career, every midwife gets a phone call where a woman says: 'I think I've broken my waters.' When this happens, we always invite them to come in and be assessed. Adele and Bert duly arrived on the ward a short time after our phone conversation.

We went through the preliminaries as usual: history, observations, and so on. They were a pleasant couple having their first baby and were naturally anxious and needing a lot of reassurance. Eventually we came to the point where we discussed an internal examination, to ensure that the baby's cord hadn't been flushed out when the membranes ruptured.

Adele was quite eager to know what was happening, although apprehensive about the procedure. During the history-taking she mentioned that she had had extensive surgery to her cervix following an abnormal pap smear. Sometimes you can feel the scar tissue on the cervix after this sort of surgery, so I was prepared for a bumpy feel.

I checked her pad when she undressed and there did seem to be a yellowish discharge present on it. It can be quite difficult at times to establish whether or not membranes have broken and her pad was no help at all; I hoped the internal would be more revealing.

I began the internal and my heart flipped. All I could feel was a large lumpy mass at the end of her vagina.

'Goodness,' I thought to myself. 'Her surgery has left her massively scarred. This cervix will never dilate enough to allow a baby out.'

Just as I was recovering from this thought, I checked my glove to see if there was evidence of any liquor draining. There was a thick creamy substance on my glove, unlike any vaginal fluid I had ever seen.

My brain went into overdrive trying to figure out what was going on with this woman. All the time, I tried to keep the expression on my face neutral so that I didn't alarm the couple, who were gazing intently at me and waiting for some intelligent comment.

Taking a deep breath, I continued my investigation and, to my eternal delight, found a protuberance among the mass that could only have been the cervix. It felt completely normal.

'So,' I thought to myself. 'What on earth is that mass that I can still feel?'

Completely bewildered, I withdrew my gloved hand, not knowing what I was going to say. Stuck to the end of my fingers was a large lump of the same creamy substance that had been on the pad. I stood gazing at my gloved hand, totally perplexed, playing with the soft lump, my brain not able to quite believe what my eyes were seeing.

Just as my thoughts coalesced into one amazing conclusion – *This looks like mashed banana* – Adele saw me looking at the substance and decided to speak.

'I've been suffering from thrush and have been using yoghurt as a treatment,' she said. (Nothing unusual about that.)

'I ran out of the plain variety and only had banana-flavoured left, so I used that.'

(Now, *that's* weird!) I was speechless – definitely something that I'm not used to being.

'I took all the large bits out first,' she added defensively. 'I heard that using yoghurt was good for thrush.'

'Yes, yes, it is,' I said, recovering momentarily and wanting to reassure her, as she looked worried. Unfortunately, the funny side of the situation, coming straight after the worry I had initially felt, was making my face contort into a grimace that was rapidly becoming uncontrollable.

I quickly mumbled an excuse and fled the delivery suite, gently closing the door.

I just as carefully closed the door to the office before collapsing into a hysterical heap at the desk, tears of laughter streaming down my face. My colleagues looked at me in amazement. It was a long time before I could compose myself sufficiently to explain my behaviour, only to begin laughing again in response to their reaction.

'How did she get it in there?' was their only comment. I had no answer for this, and I never did remember to ask her.

After I regained my self-control – delayed somewhat by another midwife walking into the office eating a banana and asking what all the fuss was about – I went back in to see Adele and Bert.

I explained to them the difficulty in positively diagnosing ruptured membranes and asked whether they would stay a while to see if more fluid became evident. Adele had obviously picked up on my amusement and wanted to talk about my views on yoghurt as a thrush treatment. We discussed the relative merits of natural versus flavoured yoghurt for quite a while.

The couple actually ended up going home and coming back in the morning for possible induction of labour, which is a normal procedure following rupture of membranes, in case of infection; 'bananaitis', in this case!

The next morning I popped my head around the door to say hello when they came in. 'The doctor will be here soon,' I said with a grin. 'He'll want to do another internal. Did you get rid of the banana?'

'Yes,' Adele replied with a definite twinkle in her eye. 'You know, I had the choice of banana or passionfruit at the time; you're probably lucky I chose the banana!'

I could only laugh along with her – the idea of passionfruit seeds was too much to imagine.

It turned out that Adele hadn't ruptured her membranes after all. She had her baby girl a week later when I was on days off. When I returned to work, one of the midwives said that my 'Banana Baby' had been born. I would have liked to see the couple again, but that's the nature of the job.

Midwives are often asked if they remember people they have cared for, or whether after a while they just all blend in with one another. Well, some are easily forgotten and others are unforgettable.

Fruit is supposed to be good for you, but in some cases . . .

The trumpets and the cavalry

NOLA AICKEN

> [Midwives] often speak of the 'incredible energy in the room' and of feeling 'drawn into the process'. It's as though the birthing woman opens a window on the universal field for others to look through, whence comes the soul of her baby.
>
> (E. Davis, *Women's Intuition*, p.28)

I was desperately missing the birth suite. What had begun as six weeks as acting clinical manager in a women's health clinic had turned into a drawn-out, four-month position. Now, at last, I was back in the maternity unit.

On a Monday in December, as the Christmas festivities were beginning, I was designated the care of Maree. I had met her several times during her pregnancy, when she had attended the antenatal clinic because of her high blood pressure. We developed an easy rapport during these visits. She was a delightful woman with three adorable children. I often looked out for them, finding them biscuits as a diversion against the monotonous hours of waiting. Maree's husband, Gary, was a staff member at the hospital.

Now in late pregnancy, Maree was admitted to the unit and was considered high risk. Her blood pressure was raised, with a reading of 140/110. It was decided by the obstetric personnel to induce her labour the next morning. I was working a morning shift on the Tuesday, so I hoped I could look after her. Continuity of care does make a difference for women *and* for midwives. It provides a wonderful opportunity for midwives to get to know the women's needs prior to the start of labour. I knew that Maree was desperate to have a good birth, because she had often taken the opportunity to talk to me about her feelings during her antenatal visits.

The following morning I arrived at seven o'clock. After the usual handover I was delegated Maree to care for during my shift. I was eager to say hello, so I headed towards her room. As I entered the room I was surprised to find that the resident doctor was already there. Amazing for 7.30 am! He was inserting an IV line, with a midwife from the night duty shift assisting.

'I wanted to start early because Maree's baby's head is still high in the pelvis. If I can't rupture the membranes I'll need to call in the obstetrician for assistance,' he said.

This early start was fine, but he seemed to have forgotten one important cog to this wheel – Maree's husband wasn't arriving until eight o'clock.

Maree was obviously anxious, but she agreed. 'You are all so busy,' she added.

It's no wonder women giving birth sometimes don't have the best experiences, when the world revolves around us and not them.

The situation didn't improve when the clinical manager then requested that I move Maree to a room in the birth suite.

'Maree, are you sure you don't want to wait for Gary to arrive?' I asked, hoping she would be assertive and suggest that we wait.

'No, you're very busy and should get started.'

I felt bad because of her generosity. Her anxiety was palpable.

Once in the birth suite, the resident doctor started the examination and I attempted to reassure Maree as best I could. I had set up the nitrous oxide mask just in case, but initially Maree didn't require it. However, as the doctor continued with the procedure, she did need a few puffs which were certainly effective. She was completely spaced out. I could sense that she was seeing at least three of me, as she smiled dreamily and tried to focus on my face.

'Take some deep breaths to clear your head, Maree!'

The doctor found the examination very difficult and couldn't rupture her membranes. Fortunately he was most professional, explaining to Maree that it would be best to contact the obstetrician to attempt the procedure. He then left the room to make the phone call, just as Gary came dashing through the door. He could have done with a parachute to pull himself up – as it was, he barely avoided slamming into the far wall. His face was a picture of confusion as he tried to take everything in.

Maree reassured Gary, as she happily waved the mask about her head. She was able to tell him that all was under control and that we were now on hold until the obstetrician arrived. He would be there 'sometime later' as he was currently 'otherwise occupied'.

From time to time I popped into the room to see how Maree and Gary were doing as they waited for the obstetrician. They were chatting quietly, trying to keep their nerves at bay.

Then, the world came to a standstill. It was close to 10 am when it actually happened. The trumpets blared. The midwives, suddenly hushed and quiet, fell back as the red carpet rolled out and He swept imperiously into the office. The One had arrived. We were ready for action.

A whispered question from the eager resident doctor came wafting from behind me: 'Have you set up the stirrups?'

'I certainly have not,' I hissed in reply. The last thing that Maree needed during her two-hour wait was to be staring at stirrups bolstered up on either side of the bed. The obstetrician would have to wait the two minutes it would take me to set them up, if indeed he chose to use stirrups at all.

Dutifully we fell into step – the obstetrician, the resident doctor and me, as we moved in single file towards Maree's room. The induction of labour would begin.

As was his usual regal custom, The One swept past the expectant father, completely ignoring him. Looking down his nose at Maree, his first words were: 'I need to carry out an examination now.'

I cut into the one-sided conversation, 'Dr (Rude), this is Maree and her husband Gary.'

'I know Maree,' came the terse reply.

Maree obediently moved to the bed, as women do, while Gary stood awkwardly in the middle of the room. I prepared the equipment while The One awaited his gloves. He then pompously sat on the side of the bed beside Maree, who was uncovered from the waist down. He was about to commence the vaginal examination.

Thump, bang, shuffle, push! The door was suddenly thrown open. The cavalry had arrived in the guise of two resident doctors. I was dumbfounded.

'WHAT ARE YOU DOING IN HERE?' the obstetrician demanded, looking over his shoulder.

I have known many to falter, to slip and to fail. Many have fallen into whimpering masses of gibbering flesh while attempting to respond to the steely-eyed look and imperial voice of The One.

The boldest resident, a slip of a thing with immaculate blonde hair, answered without even a twitch to her body. 'We're interested in observing the procedure. We heard there is a high head and that's obviously unusual.'

(I visualised a lonesome head sailing around the ceiling of the room, and the three resident doctors raising their eyes to the heavens in awe.)

I didn't wait for The One to speak first. 'No!' I called out. 'Maree is apprehensive enough, and it's not appropriate to have three of you in the room.'

This situation reminded me of the old days, when students lined labour ward walls to observe all sorts of procedures performed on women, never caring to ask their permission or consider their right to privacy.

But the cheeky little resident wasn't to be outdone by

a mere midwife. She mooched over to Maree and ducked her head close. 'Can we all stay, pleeeaaasssse? We can learn from this,' she sweetly begged.

Maree replied: 'Yes, it's alright for you to stay,' at the same moment as I mumbled 'No, it's *not* alright!'

'YOU DO NOT ALL NEED TO BE HERE!'

The One had spoken.

'IF YOU HAVE SEEN THIS TYPE OF EXAMINATION BEFORE, YOU CAN GO.'

The mooching resident moved to Maree's left side, knowing she had done well. She glanced at me through fluttering lids as if to say, 'I'm staying and you can't do anything about it.' The other resident sidled quietly along the wall and slipped out of the room.

I encouraged Gary to find a place by Maree's right side, knowing that if he didn't move in soon, he might be outdone for a space by the enthusiastic cavalry.

The One moved easily into teaching mode, his deep voice rumbling with his vast obstetrical knowledge. 'I would normally attempt a difficult ROM with the woman's legs in stirrups; however, we will try without for the present.'

So, he began. I handed him the Amnihook. He wasn't able to rupture the membranes, so he asked for the Alligators. A great gush of liquor spread over the sheets and on to the bed, a slow cascade of fluid dripping to the floor. The appropriate oohs and aahs were heard from the gathered cavalry, signalling the success of The One. He then checked that babe's head was presenting. I could establish from his expression that the head was where it should be, and not floating bodiless above us.

The One then requested a scalp electrode. I thought he was a brave man indeed to attempt to attach an electrode to a mobile head and a cervix dilated to only 3 centimetres!

Not to be outdone in his moment of glory, though, he dexterously swung the electrode in the direction of babe's head, who I imagined would be creeping higher in an attempt to avoid the cruel twist of the electrode into its scalp.

The silence of concentration ensued. *I think I can. I think I can.*

But he wasn't successful after all, and suggested we attach the abdominal CTG and start the trace. Anticipating his inability to attach the electrode, I was already organising this.

It was all over. The cavalry left the room as noisily as they had entered.

Without looking at either Maree or Gary, The One's last words as he left the room were: 'Sit her up as soon as possible to assist the baby's head to move down.' Then he was gone.

I changed Maree's bed linen and made her comfortable. She sat up in the bed and I finished attaching the CTG. Listening to the continuous *dub dub* sound of her babe's heartbeat made her feel much less stressed.

I felt confident leaving Maree and Gary while I prepared the Syntocinon for the second phase of the induction.

'Can I go to the loo before you start?' Maree asked when I returned.

We disconnected the CTG lines and the IVT connections and our little procession shuffled in unison to the toilet. I reassured Maree about the Syntocinon and told her that I wouldn't hurry its titration, that we would allow her body to adjust as she progressed in labour. She was relieved.

The babe's heart rate continued its happy little *dub dub* sound on the CTG, not at all worried by the Syntocinon running through Maree's veins in an attempt to move it from the safe world it had known for many months.

Maree's sister Rose had travelled from Melbourne to be at the birth. A knock at the door heralded her arrival. Initially giggly at the prospect of being a part of this experience, she overwhelmed the room with her excitement. She didn't have children herself, so this was a real adventure. I felt a touch uneasy with her laughter and gaiety, and hoped she would settle into serious mode once the contractions intensified.

Maree was now concentrating intensely. She was magnificent to watch and I was impressed as she took each contraction as it came with confidence and courage. I knew she could do this. I could see that she would make every effort to get through the experience herself. Gary was wonderfully supportive, but as he wasn't required at her side completely as yet, he sat by the table with a coffee in hand.

Soon after midday I noted that Maree was concentrating much more seriously with her contractions, closing her eyes and breathing through. *Fuuff-huh-fuuff-huh.*

Rose was chatting, chatting, endlessly chatting.

Fuuff-huh-fuuff-huh-fuuff-shhhhhhhhhhhhooosh. Maree turned to Rose at the finish of one intense contraction and gasped: 'Please don't talk until I finish the contraction!'

'We need to support Maree by being quiet during her contractions,' I explained to Rose, 'so that she can focus on what she's doing.'

Fortunately Rose took the cues. 'Can I massage your feet, then?'

An excellent idea, I thought. I placed the portable screen around the entrance of the door to ensure privacy. It always seems to happen that the crowd and the cavalry outside forget to knock and wait for permission to enter during the most crucial, private times of a woman's labour and birth. It's as if a signal goes off to all and sundry out there to come into the birth room for reasons that aren't always apparent. Once, for instance, I was catching a baby. As I turned slightly on hearing the *shhh-bang* sound of a closing door, I was thumped in the ribs by an attacking meal tray.

'Lunch?' the domestic asked meekly, as her eyes slid to the naked woman and the birthing baby before her.

'Not now!' I replied.

Or the *shhh-bang* as the notorious jug lady stands in the middle of the room while a very private vaginal examination is being carried out, saying: 'Where do you want me to put this?'

'Well, certainly not where my hand is right now!' comes the angry response.

Or *shhh-bang* – the medical cavalry charging in, loudly discussing the recent incident of Mrs H in theatre following a manual removal: '. . . She bled like stormwater in a drainpipe! Lucky for her she was in hospital . . .' All eyes suddenly look over at the woman, lying with the sheets pulled back while I'm changing a pad.

Shhh-bang! The endless saga of the midwife looking for the lost keys. 'Do you have the keys?' the midwife whines. 'Mandy said she gave them to you a while back. I've checked with positively eevveerryone else. Oh, sorrrrry, I didn't realise you were in the middle of a vaginal examination!'

Shhh-bang!

When Maree returned from the toilet again – lines up, commence procession and shuffle – everyone found their positions in the circle of support. I was excited to see this happening. With a strong circle of support, a woman will get through the glass darkly, because she is surrounded by those who love her the most.

Gary found his calling with Maree's back. As each contraction assailed her body, he valiantly massaged the area that most needed rubbing. Gary also placed a hot pack on other parts of her back. Rose sat at Maree's feet, massaging them skilfully hour after hour after hour. The little circle worked together to help Maree achieve what she most fervently wanted – a beautiful birth.

I felt Maree still had a little way to go, but I believed that her babe's head was moving down into the pelvis. This was exciting news, but unfortunately I wasn't able to maintain continuous monitoring. With Syntocinon running, I needed to know exactly what her baby was doing. I notified the resident to come.

Enter the resident. She briskly carried out the vaginal examination and efficiently placed the scalp electrode on the baby's head. It was a simple procedure now with the baby further down in the pelvis and Maree's cervix more dilated. The resident thought that Maree was about 4–5 centimetres; reasonably good progress, considering the babe's head still needed to move down on to the cervix.

Now with a good trace on the baby, I felt I should 'up' the Syntocinon to encourage the contractions to become a little stronger. I discussed this with Maree, who agreed. Within minutes she was feeling fragile with the intensified contractions.

'Maree, would you like to try leaning over a beanbag?'

'Anything!' came the terse response.

The forward position was excellent for her. When she moved over on to the beanbag, Gary found the back massage easier, while Rose stayed with her successful foot massage. We were on a roll! I prepared the equipment for birth and continued monitoring Maree's progress. With the teamwork happening, I only needed to reassure Maree every now and then and observe events. I didn't want the momentum in the room to change, so I skipped lunch.

Maree was working hard with the contractions by the time Judy, the afternoon midwife, came on to take over from me. However, she still had incredible control and I felt so proud of her efforts – she was brilliant. Despite rolling, intense contractions, she had requested no pain relief.

She sat on the side of the bed for several contractions, leaning into Gary, and I noted a flood of bloodstained liquor. The baby's heart rate was fine, but I asked her to move back on to the bed so that I could check that all was okay. I stopped the Syntocinon and continued to observe the CTG. With the next contraction the loss had settled, so it was obviously a gush of liquor with some bloodstaining from positive progress.

It was now close to 3 pm and I was in a quandary as to whether I should go or stay. I was due to finish my shift at 3.15 pm. Maree was close to second stage, unsettled, sweating and shaking, and her contractions were bumper to bumper – sure signs of late first stage.

I was in a dilemma. There was no reason for me to stay, other than my desire to be part of this special event.

I finally decided to go. Wishing Maree all the best with a warm hug, I told Gary and Rose how wonderful they were, too, and I then left. I knew they would be okay in Judy's capable hands.

My curiosity eventually got the better of me later that night, and I rang the unit at 7 pm. 'Maree had a baby boy at four minutes to 4 pm without a hitch!' said Judy with jubilation. 'She had a tiny tear, too small to mention, and a wonderful birth!'

Maree must surely be so proud. She had achieved the birth that she so wished to have. Her courage had helped her make it through the labour. Maree's high-risk status had meant that interventions would happen and yet she still managed to have a lovely birth. Her circle of strength, Gary and Rose, were indeed a team to be reckoned with as they supported her.

I could imagine that Maree would have birthed with an exhilaration that not many women in the high-risk category manage to achieve these days.

Joseph Gary was born, all 9lb 10 oz of him! What an achievement! What a birth!

Funny peculiar

A. E. MOATES

It started to drizzle as I stepped carefully among the animal droppings. As I put my heavy load down, I thought what a strange sort of day it was. Even the rainbow that split the horizon seemed to leer at me in a parody of a smile. Over the years, I'd witnessed life-and-death struggles and watched families transform with the arrival of a new baby. There had been happy times, frustrating days, sad situations, and moments of revelation amid routine. It was a peculiar day – a funny peculiar kind of day. And it wasn't anything to do with Gizelle finally asking for help.

I first met Gizelle and her husband Brian a few days before she had her first baby. She was to be induced at

37 weeks, but this was something she had little interest in. Brian, on the other hand, seemed determined to ask everyone about what would happen, and how he could play a major role in making it happen. He worked somewhere on the fringes of the healthcare industry as a sales rep for a large chemical company, so he felt qualified to manage the coming event.

Gizelle didn't seem to mind the waiting. She didn't have the worries and distractions that age invited, despite the fact that her first pregnancy was proving troublesome. Incessant vomiting had been her constant companion for the first twenty weeks or so. Now she was in hospital because at 32 weeks her waters had broken. With each passing day, Gizelle moved a little closer to her destiny of motherhood with a serene, restrained countenance, which counterbalanced perfectly with her husband's manic behaviour.

At the time, I was having second thoughts about becoming a midwife. I'd spent my first rotation as a student midwife in the postnatal area, trying not to get in the way. Once the unit manager accused me of hiding behind closed curtains and she wasn't far off the mark, but her comment was unjustified, as I was trying desperately to get a baby to latch on and breastfeed – a case of trying to fit a square peg in a round hole. My idea of midwifery had been smiling women wearing pink bed jackets, and sitting up in bed nursing tiny little bundles. But the reality had been brutal. The tiny little bundles were lively and loud, not to mention their mums. That's not to say it was always like that, but there were times when it overwhelmed me.

So, it was with guarded relief that I crossed the floor, literally, to get some serenity. I was doing my first antenatal rotation. Not a baby in sight, and the noise was subdued. My allocated beds housed a variety of antenatal complaints that involved taking regular observations of mother and foetus. One of my patients was Gizelle. We were of a similar age, yet she seemed a world apart from me in all other respects.

'What's that you're doing?' Brian asked when I arrived at Gizelle's bedside with the blood-pressure machine. He stood behind me and watched the procedure intently, and expressed disappointment when I declined to take his blood pressure. Fortunately, Gizelle had normal readings.

'How are you feeling today?' I asked her.

'She's had a good day, but I'm still getting bouts of nausea,' Brian replied. 'And I think I'm getting a haemorrhoid now!' He was looking at me far too hopefully – and I was certainly not going to confirm or deny his suspicion.

'I think I have an enema to see to,' I said, escaping.

Over the next few days my encounters with Gizelle and Brian continued. Gizelle never contradicted anything Brian said, nor expressed any interest in what was happening to her or her body. At times I suspected it was only the spectre of Gizelle who rested in that bed, and her physical body floated somewhere above the stratosphere, with Brian tugging her strings like a marionette.

Her baby was growing well in utero, and her waters seeped rather than leaked.

As a student midwife I was expected to observe a certain number of deliveries before working in the delivery area. One day, by some stroke of strange fortune, I was the only student around and was introduced to the mysteries of childbirth. By that same quirk of fortune, it was the birth of Gizelle's first boy which I was compelled to witness.

'Get the bloody thing outa me, will ya!' Gizelle yelled. She made me leap backwards even though everyone else ignored her.

'Just pant – *ph, ph, ph*,' crooned the midwife. I all but panted myself.

'Push!' screeched Brian. I tried.

The obstetrician didn't have anything to say. His head was hidden between Gizelle's knees. For some reason her legs were in stirrups. I hovered somewhere near her left foot, which was almost at my eye-level, as Gizelle writhed and tried to break free. Something poked me in the back and I jerked forward. The charge nurse of the delivery area was pushing me forward. She seemed to enjoy the look of utter horror on my face. It may be absurd, but I don't like the sight of blood, and there seemed to be a copious amount of it flooding about Gizelle. As I stumbled forward I knocked the obstetrician further into Gizelle's nether regions. I fully expected to hear a pop when he suddenly wrenched his head away from Gizelle's knees and looked straight through me.

'Keep out of my way,' he said.

And that's how I came to be involved on the periphery of Gizelle's family life.

Gizelle, after her surprising outburst, lay back, exhausted but essentially back to her disinterested self. Brian was busy earbashing the obstetrician, quizzing him about the tensile strength of the sutures that were being expertly inserted at about five a minute. There seemed to be rather a lot and I would know, since I was allocated the suture scissors to cut them as directed. Behind me the now-familiar newborn baby cry was diverting, but not so much so that I risked incurring the obstetrician's wrath. A midwife was bustling about the room, jangling metal kidney dishes containing syringes and vials, slamming cupboard doors and talking about the beautiful spring day outside.

By another peculiar quirk of fate, the antenatal situation became extremely quiet and I was forced to revisit the postnatal ward for a few days, and had the pleasure of looking after Gizelle and her new baby. In terms of quality care, the exercise was pointless, sincc I was a novice. Yet it was commendable, in the era of fractured care, that she was getting some continuity of care. Having the same carer didn't make much impact, however. My help seemed redundant – Gizelle remained in her stratosphere and seemed unaware that I was the same staff member who had been hanging around for days.

Brian, however, was very aware, and very punctilious about how punctilious I was with the care of his son first, his wife second, and him a chivalrous third. He was still hinting about his haemorrhoids. I, apologetically, seemed to have an inordinate number of urgent enemas to attend to.

Graduation came and went. I had a photo to prove it. We all seemed happy enough, certainly on the day, and some of us got tipsy on the night. There were a few vacancies in the unit and I was offered one of them. At the time I didn't have anything better to do, so I accepted and began my life as a midwife, rotating through antenatal, postnatal, delivery suite and special care nursery.

Being allocated the first-time mother inductions had in itself seemed a cruel initiation for me. It was the norm to put in the hard hours, seeing the first hopeful, exciting, tremulous bravado of the women vowing not to seek pain relief, smiling through the first contractions, then clawing at me as they demanded an epidural – 'Now! NOW, do you hear?!' – then miss the delivery itself, which usually happened a few hours after my shift ended.

There were compensations, and some memorable experiences. There seemed to be a lot of boys being born that year, and not everyone clawed at me. Yes, delivery suite had put the dot on the 'i' for me. My ultimate destiny didn't lie in delivering babies, but at the time it was reward enough to continue.

My first year as a fully fledged midwife stomped onwards. So, it wasn't an absolute quirk of fate that I happened to come to work one hot summer morning and found myself allocated to look after a young mother just about to deliver her baby. Brian remembered me, but Gizelle just gazed about, not really catching my eye. I told myself that it was because she was in labour and shouldn't be expected to reminisce about our previous encounter. Not long after I arrived, the obstetrician arrived. He was in a hurry to hurry things along.

'Just do it!' Gizelle said. She scratched and clawed and screamed and let go of some of her serenity, especially when the pudendal block anaethesia was needled in. A student midwife stood uncertainly by the bed waiting for the inevitable and trying to avoid being thumped by Gizelle's feet, which were swinging wildly around in stirrups. I buzzed to let another midwife know it was time to come in and receive the baby. The ergometrine vial had been checked and waited in the syringe for me to administer once the obstetrician directed me. The forceps clanged as the obstetrician lined them up visually – like a master chef with a pair of salad spoons. Brian seemed disappointed when denied the opportunity to pull out the baby – Gizelle's second boy. He cried. The baby did, too.

Unfortunately, there were complications in the form of retained placental tissue and a subsequent haemorrhage, and Gizelle was rushed off to the operating theatre. Brian stayed and helped me give his latest son his first bath. There was lots to discuss. Issues about the first baby, and hints that maybe Brian's haemorrhoids were threatening an exacerbation in effect. There was no alternative but to listen and reply vaguely, and ask the odd distracting question.

'How is Gizelle?' I asked. According to Brian, Gizelle never really had much to say most of the time.

'How about the family?' There was something Brian couldn't disclose, but the short version was that Gizelle's family didn't want anything to do with Brian.

Then the baby started to cry, and it was time to tip out the bathwater.

I visited Gizelle the next day. It was good PR. She looked at me in a vague, disinterested way. I restrained myself from giving her a résumé about how I'd seen both her boys born and wasn't it a coincidence – maybe a good one! Whether she lacked capacity or chose to remain aloof was a mystery to me. There seemed little point in labouring the issue, so I said goodbye and good luck. She didn't need my help.

There is some point in most people's lives when time seems to move along in top gear. For me, study, marriage and more study seemed to blur with the seasons. I continued to rotate through the midwifery areas, getting classified as a Clinical Nurse Specialist in midwifery, but I preferred to work in the special care nursery. The years had finely honed my nursing passion. I loved working with babies. It didn't matter that some were tiny, many were sick – all were special and beautiful in a memorable way.

So, it wasn't surprising that I was working when I met Gizelle's third boy. He was wheeled in via the portable incubator from the operating theatre. Like the first two, he was vitally robust, merely boarding briefly until his mother returned from the operating theatre. Brian trailed in after his baby, engaged in a deep one-sided monologue with the paediatrician.

'What are the odds of a baby getting into the breech position just days before the due date?' he was saying. 'And what's the record for the number of times a cord can wrap around a baby's neck?'

Gizelle's return to the ward was delayed due to a problem with the anaesthetic, so we had the pleasure of her baby's company, and Brian's, for a few hours. It was déjà vu that found Brian and me matched up to bath his baby.

Times were more enlightened now and we did let the

mum do this if she desired. I'd even suggested waiting until Gizelle returned, but Brian demurred, saying: 'I do all the baby care.'

Uncharacteristically, he seemed to run out of things to say as I towelled the baby dry. We'd covered the topics of toilet-training and bedwetting, and I'd skilfully skirted any mention of haemorrhoids. Gizelle, it seems, exercised no discipline over her sons' behaviour, and Brian wasn't so comfortable in being a liberal parent. It could have been the lighting cast by an early autumn sunset, but perhaps the grey that peppered his hair was new since our last encounter; his features were certainly becoming gaunt.

Later I watched in incomprehension as Gizelle looked at me but failed to acknowledge our past associations. Her latest baby lay snug in the crook of her arm.

'Hello. It's me. Again!' I laughed, but Gizelle didn't respond. It was as if we were strangers. I felt deflated. Obviously my participation in some small way with the arrival of her three sons didn't seem particularly unusual to her. Nor did she note my own advanced state of pregnancy. But why would she? There wasn't any bond. There never had been. I'd not been helpful or illuminating in any appreciative way. Gizelle didn't need my help.

'Does he have to stay here with me?' Gizelle asked, and I wasn't sure if she was talking about the baby or Brian.

My priorities changed with the birth of my own baby. Mothering duties weren't particularly onerous, but they were time-consuming. For a while I worked part-time. Along with the part-time work I developed some paranoia. It seemed that part-time work equated with a half-time brain. While still passionate about babies, my involvement became more like care-taking, and therefore was unsatisfactory to me. So I took my half-time brain, studied full-time for a year, and then started looking for work as a maternal and child health nurse.

Many years ago I'd tagged along with my mother when she took my infant brother to the infant welfare nurse. That nurse had seemed so wise and knowing. Mum always seemed impressed by her depth of knowledge and encouraged by her wisdom. Yet this aura seemed to elude me, at least in how I felt about my ability to be wise and knowledgeable. At first I did relief work as well as my midwifery work. My own little baby had grown into a toilet-trained toddler and I hoped that my firsthand experiences would give me an empathic edge.

It was a kind mentor who helped me to achieve my first regular maternal and child health nurse position in a semi-rural area. The families I worked with were practical and pragmatic. Whether I was ever more than a sounding board for them to air their concerns and grievances about the challenge of mothering, I don't know. Whether I had become wise with time is doubtful. But it was during this sojourn that I had my final encounter with Gizelle.

One grey late winter morning I collected the new birth notices from the council. One of them notified me that a woman, whose first name was Gizelle, had recently given birth to a boy. I didn't recognise the surname, so I didn't think it was the same Gizelle I'd encountered previously. I called her. The phone distorts the voice a little, so I wasn't sure if it was her and she certainly didn't seem to recognise my name.

'Yes, you can visit if you want to. I'm not going anywhere,' she said.

The sun was trying to warm the day when I left the centre just after midday. Rain was forecast and clouds were galloping up the treed horizon. I checked the Melways – Gizelle lived on the outskirts of the village.

The car lurched over deep water-filled potholes and my windscreen wipers smeared mud across the glass. Gizelle's house sat snugly behind a paling fence which gave substantial glimpses of patchy grass. A number of water-logged steps reached up to the front door.

I put on my professional poise.

My first knock wasn't heard, but I could hear the distant murmur of voices, so I knocked again for longer, almost bruising my knuckles in the process. The murmurs continued but seemed to come closer. Gizelle peered around the opening door.

'Hello, Gizelle!'

'You must be the nurse,' she said. She didn't seem to remember me. Maybe it was because I was wearing casual clothes rather than a uniform. Perhaps there was sun glare in her eyes, even though it wasn't very sunny. Or maybe it was too much effort to try. She looked a bit pale and drawn, and she had streaks of grey in her fringe.

'Congratulations on the birth of your baby boy,' I said, trying to sound assured. But I didn't feel very confident standing there in her doorway. I was missing Brian already. Was he lurking inside somewhere?

'I've got four boys. My fiancé has three, plus a girl.'

'Fiancé?'

'His kids come on weekends. It's very messy on weekends,' she said, looking around.

I looked, too. I'd edged my way into what was obviously meant to be a parlour, but was crammed with various pieces of furniture and four enormous washing baskets overflowing with clothes.

Gizelle was more vocal than I'd ever known her to be. Brian had been ditched. (Something about too much talking, which she couldn't stand anymore, and hadn't her family warned her about him?) Besides, she was now very much in love with her fiancé, who, like her, was divorced, and ecstatic that their love had been sealed with the birth of a son.

It didn't seem the same without Brian, somehow, but there was certainly something different about Gizelle. Indeed, the latest baby was as healthy as all her others, only bigger. He wanted to breastfeed all the time.

'I have to get *him* his lunch. He likes Vegemite sandwiches. Will you hold *him* while I make them?' she said as she shoved her baby at me. The first *him*, being boy number three, poked the other *him* in my arms. I don't think he cared much for his new brother, and grinned when the baby cried. While trying to soothe the baby and deter him from rooting at my breast, I wandered about the room and suddenly sneezed.

There was a strong smell of detergent emanating from the washing baskets. And was that steam rising from them?

Gizelle returned with a plateful of carefully cut sandwiches. She gave them to the young boy, then took the baby away from me and began to feed him. She seemed very focused and confident in her manner.

'You must be very busy now,' I said.

'Yes. I never have enough time. There's always so much to do.'

Perhaps domesticity had caught up with Gizelle. Then I had a light-bulb moment. It wasn't a spectre of Gizelle who was telling me about the realities of her life. It was Gizelle herself. She'd come down from the stratosphere and had started to live. Deep inside, I wished the same for Brian.

'Well, I'm here to help,' I said sincerely. Sometimes it's not what you know, or how you come to know it, that's important. It's what you can do and how you do it.

And I knew exactly what I was going to do.

The brown sheep nudged me as I moved around the clothesline. There was a white one on the periphery butting his brown friend. There were ducks and chickens, and three rabbits, too. As I finished pegging out all the clothes from the first steaming washing basket and started on the second, I chuckled to myself. It was a funny day. Funny peculiar.

Names have been changed to protect confidentiality.

FROM WAR ZONES to the BUSH

Women's business

JENNIFER RICHMOND

Out there in the 1970s, the red earth was as hard as iron, except for the top layer of dust, fine as orange talcum powder, blowing up in choking clouds to get in under nappies, into noses, ears, eyes and mouths. Babies' mouths. And the sun was rough and stinging, scorching the land barren. Shade was sparse. The Aboriginal camps were a series of industrial-sized breezeways to make the most of any stirring of the air, despite the bulldust. And the flies.

I brushed the flies away from baby Betty who at two weeks of age was losing weight, but certainly not from anorexia. Betty was screaming her dissatisfaction: the little singlet she'd bulged out of just a week ago wrinkled now. Her loosely wrapped bunny rug was smudged dust-red. I looked at her mother, Rosie, a plump, passive teenager in a stretchy yellow sundress. We walked slowly towards the shade of the clinic so that I, a midwife for less than two years, could think.

At fifteen or so, Rosie married an older man, Colin. By older, I mean late fifties. This type of marriage was commonplace. As an Elder it was expected that Colin would take a second wife to care for him and his first wife in their old age. But Colin's first wife wasn't pleased to take the pretty, but rather simple, Rosie into the camp. Seemed like just another child, certainly not a help; not another pair of hands, but another mouth to feed. The other women of the camp sided with Colin's first wife. So, Colin, a man of power and authority, found himself helpless when Rosie took to trailing around after him, instead of staying in the camp and doing women's work. And the other women just got more and more annoyed with Rosie.

Unfortunately, Rosie's mothercraft advice was expected to come from her new family. Now she was married, there was no taking the dusty track back to her mother Clara's camp. Not that Rosie gave any hint of wanting to return, although Clara's campfire burned, just visible in the flat landscape, about a kilometre away.

While it wouldn't have been forbidden for Rosie to visit her mother, it was taboo for Clara to approach Colin's camp, and I had a sneaking suspicion that Rosie's mother was pleased to have married off her 'slow' daughter.

Clara herself was an Elder, high up in women's business. She had enough on her plate, with tribal business, all her other kids and a sick husband. She still had a child on the breast. A child every couple of years.

Although she'd only be in her late thirties she had weary eyes and shoulders; large but drooping breasts. Hard enough to do even the essential things with an unreliable water supply and a mixture of town and bush food. There might only be wallaby to throw on the campfire, fur and all, for tea. Or a fat goanna sizzling in the embers.

So, Rosie's place was at Colin's camp. And when she became pregnant, word had it that Colin was pleased – he liked little kids, and maybe he thought it would stop Rosie bothering him when he was occupied with men's business.

When I could find Rosie I gave her antenatal care and tried to pass on some mothercraft. But unlike the other first-time mothers, Rosie just sat under the healthy food groups poster in the clinic, slow-eyed and dreamy. She was strong and healthy enough, but I wondered how she would manage the demands of a baby. I told myself that good postnatal care would see us through.

Sure enough, things didn't start well. The district hospital was a place where people went to die, wasn't it? In an era when first-time mothers stayed in hospital for six days postpartum, the frightened Rosie took her baby home as soon as she'd had a sleep and a good feed. The day after a normal labour and delivery of a healthy 4.5-kilogram daughter she left the hospital, got a lift out of town on the back of a ute heading for Colin's camp.

The other families clustered under the industrial tin roof were excited by the new baby's arrival, and for a while all grievances were put aside. These people were happy celebrating a new life in their group. The women coo-ed, while the little kids fingered Betty's perfect hands and face in awe, leaving grimy fingerprints on her cotton hospital layette.

Before the second postnatal visit, news came to me of Rosie and baby Betty. In the clinic, William, the Aboriginal health worker, told me: 'You gotta do something about that baby Betty. All the families are complaining it's cryin' all the day and all the night. Nobody got any rest. Even that Colin, he gone out bush to get away from the noise.'

At Colin's camp Rosie toed the dust, but the other women had plenty to say.

'She's not feedin' it enough!'

'That baby Betty cries so loud they can hear her way in town.'

'She got no milk for that baby.'

'That baby's cryin' 'cause it hasn't got no tucker.'

Now, in the clinic, Rosie and I looked at Betty. She did look hungry. Rosie looked at the floor and whispered, 'Sister, I want to feed 'im with the bottles like the ladies at the hospital.'

My ears curled. Artificial feeding in developing-world conditions puts the baby at grave risk. But Rosie had made up her mind and wouldn't put the baby to the breast. She shook her head when I told her that Betty would get sick without her mother's milk. Not even a description of all the work involved in cleaning and making up formula would change Rosie's mind.

And how would they keep the formula chilled?

She didn't know.

William had an idea.

'Colin can get that old generator going. Then they can get a fridge for all them bottles.'

So, it was agreed. Right there in the clinic, Rosie had her first lesson in making up formula from the emergency supplies in the top cupboard.

'Wash your hands, Rosie. With the soap.'

Betty's suck was strong and so determined, that even with fine holes in the teat, she guzzled down that bottle and went straight to satisfied sleep. When I showed Rosie how to get Betty's wind up, a lazy burp oozed out of the lolling baby mouth. The little kids watching giggled, and Rosie hugged Betty like she'd never let her go. The silence was heavenly.

The mysterious but efficient bush telegraph recalled Colin. He sidled into camp from the outstation late that morning with three young men in cowboy hats. They got to work on the generator that had lain stripped down by a dry petrol pump all the months I'd been visiting. By the end of the day a brand-new bar fridge stood on the cement slab in Colin's camp and Rosie had been to the chemist in town. She came home in a battered, dust-covered Holden, low to the ground with baby-feeding equipment, every item on the list crossed off. Finally, an old metal meat safe kept flies and grimy little fingers away from the baby's things.

I wish I could say that peace reigned. Betty was finally quiet, but thanks to the generator the camp soon bristled with ghetto blasters playing country music, and a makeshift TV aerial was hoisted like a metal flag. All this to the steady spatter of the generator, but no one complained now. And despite my misgivings, Betty gained weight quickly and metamorphosed into a personality as placid as her mother.

By the weekend, Rosie had to fly solo with the bottles.

The temporary truce of the homecoming was over and the other women called her lazy, said she had to do this for herself. For Betty. And maybe Rosie *was* a little lazy, or just too young, or too slow. Maybe they'd relent and lend a hand . . .

Anyway, for the first time she was on her own.

I left for town with a final word of advice: 'Wash your hands, Rosie. Remember to wash your hands first with the soap. And keep the flies away.'

'Yes, Sister,' whispered Rosie.

On Monday morning the camp was eerily quiet: no generator hum, only Betty's wailing.

William filled me in. 'Generator broke down and Betty got the diarrhoea.'

Hungry now, a little dehydrated and sick. Her temperature was up.

While Betty was in hospital, Rosie and Colin camped in town. And while they were away, life returned to Colin's camp. There was no more country music but the old men were singing, women walked with a spring in their step, even the dogs curled up happily in the dust or ran around in a big mob like the kids.

When Betty's return was imminent, I drove past Colin's camp with William with a heavy heart. I knew what would happen when the baby came home: recurrent diarrhoea, eye and ear infections, cough, failure to thrive, lots of crying. The bush worked against a bottle-fed babe.

William read my mind but smiled enigmatically. In an annoyingly superior way he said, 'Don't worry, Sister Jenny. Everything be alright soon.'

That day and the next there was a lot of traffic on the track. Old Holdens cloaked in red dust took carloads of women up and down. I gazed down to Clara's camp. The hot wind brought the sound of women singing. Business was being transacted, women's business.

Betty came home on Rosie's hip the bonny babe she was meant to be. In hospital she had started to smile, and Rosie was brimming with confidence.

Next day my first stop was Colin's camp, but Betty wasn't there, nor was Rosie. They waved me down to Clara's camp, laughing at my surprise. As my vehicle threw up clouds of orange bulldust I wondered what was afoot – no generator down there. First thing I saw was Rosie in her yellow stretchy dress, seated under the bough shelter with the other women and little kids. Beaming, she waved me over. And there was Betty, happy as Larry, fixed to the breast of her wet nurse: Clara.

Later, curious, I asked Clara what made her agree to take on Betty when she had every reason not to, not the least of which was a baby of her own still on the breast.

She smiled that tired smile and looked at her calloused hands.

'Well, Sister, I tell you true. Couldn't stand no more of that mob up there complaining.'

Hard labour

HEATHER HARRIS

I am working for a relief organisation – Medecins Sans Frontières – in a war zone, living in an isolated part of northern Sri Lanka where civil war has raged for over twenty years.

Thousands of internally displaced people are fleeing the fighting further north, stretching the rural hospital's resources to breaking point. Although it has about 130 rickety beds, it usually houses double that number of patients, and by the time each patient's bystander is squeezed in, there is little room to move around. We are there as part of an expatriate team augmenting the surgical and obstetric program, run by five nurses and five midwives. My job is to run an education program for the untrained workers who staff the place – people whose nursing abilities are astonishing. They perform most of the complicated procedures – dressings, cannulations, catheterisation, resuscitation – you name, they do it.

I work in Maternity as well. The national midwives here often work an eighteen-hour day, so they take a rest when they can. The labour room is a dishevelled affair with three beds along one wall separated by spectacularly inadequate old curtains. With about 130 babies born every month, these beds are rarely empty.

This day dawns bright, hot and dusty. Fritz, our expat obstetrician, is going away on four days' R&R. He should have left at 7 am so that they can pass through the army checkpoint early and cross into the cleared area and freedom, but when I arrive for breakfast at 7.30 am I see the four-wheel drive is still here. Fritz has been up until 2 am dealing with obstetric emergencies. He looks exhausted and worried, knowing he is leaving behind a ward full of complicated cases. There are two other doctors here – Andre, a young Belgian surgeon, and Marina, an Austrian anaesthetist. Neither has any obstetric experience, however.

'I'm happy to do any surgery you might need, but you will have to make the obstetric decisions,' Andre says to me. Until Fritz rejoins us Tuesday evening, I am now part of the obstetric team, and I feel the gentle weight of that responsibility settle upon my shoulders.

I walk down the dusty track to the hospital. It is buzzing – partly from busyness and partly from flies. Marina and I make the ward round. Here lies a woman looking very ill; pale, sweaty and retching into a makeshift vomit bowl. Yesterday she'd had a hydatidiform mole removed and is hypovolaemic. Her pulse is rapid, her blood pressure low. Marina orders another IV be inserted and we start her on Hartman's, a solution that will help to correct any fluid or electrolyte imbalance.

Inside the labour ward the three beds are occupied. The bed nearest the door holds a young woman at the end of her second pregnancy. Three years before, during her first labour, her baby had become distressed and had died before birth despite an emergency Caesarean being done. This pregnancy, we have brought her to sit in hospital for her last few weeks and watch over her while her belly swells. Her baby's heart is checked every day. She is bored with doing nothing, but she sits around patiently, and her baby grows.

Then without warning yesterday, when we listened for her foetal heart . . . nothing. Total silence. That eerie no-sound you get when life has gone from the womb.

No vibrancy, no kicks, no reassuring *thud-thud*.

Just a few crackles . . . and nothing more.

So, Fritz has had no choice but to induce her labour before he left. He has given her one of the precious prostoglandin tablets we have, to start her contractions. She lies there, sadly, waiting for the inevitable, knowing there will be no joy today. It is a potentially dangerous situation as she already has a scar on her uterus. We don't want to cause a rupture by inducing her too aggressively, nor do we want her to endure another Caesarean section to deliver another dead baby. A two-unit Syntocinon infusion hangs at her bed, dripping slowly in the oppressive heat.

Next to her lies a woman with a foetal bradycardia and now over 42 weeks pregnant. She is labouring, but not strongly. Her waters have broken and the fluid is clear. We have a Syntocinon drip slowly running to strengthen the contractions but the situation is fraught, and I urge our wonderful Sri Lankan midwife, Karmela, to keep a close ear on her foetal heart. Dear Karmela with the soft brown eyes, kindly face and a lifetime of midwifery experience. A true *sage femme*.

In the third bed lies a woman with a borderline high blood pressure, another Syntocinon drip running and about 2–3 centimetres dilated. They lie quietly together in this crowded, hot, claustrophobic room, waiting for what the day will bring. Their dark brown skins glisten with sweat, their black eyes anxious. Their bystanders wait outside, sitting patiently in the shade and fanning themselves. All patients have a person who comes into hospital with them and stays with them constantly. The bystander attends to all the basic needs of the patient, from washing to feeding, and it's unthinkable not to have one.

We continue the ward round, ordering haemoglobin tests, the occasional malaria test. All the tiny babies – there are six under 2 kilograms – are progressing well. They lie snuggled beside their mothers, sleeping in the heat, naso-gastric tubes taped to their tiny wizened faces, and a large plastic bottle of hot water wrapped in an old sari tucked in beside them to maintain their temperature. Some are shielded with a netting food cover so that the flies won't annoy them, but not everyone can afford such a luxury. I have a special interest in infant feeding, so these babies are *my* 'babies' and I take great joy in watching them grow. At least they are all doing well.

At 11 am three women arrive from transfer. The first is bleeding from an incomplete miscarriage. She is stable but will need a curette. Arrangements are made and she is wheeled off to the operating theatre. The second *tangachchi* (young woman) is a shyly smiling eighteen-year-old from a village further east, who stands only 138 centimetres tall – she literally fits underneath my armpit! Tiny and bulging at term with her first pregnancy, she's not in labour, but has come to wait until her baby decides it is ready to greet the world. I palpate her abdomen and feel the baby's head overlapping her pubic bone.

'No way will that head fit through that pelvis,' I think to myself. But we'll wait and see . . .

The third woman is contracting and draining meconium-stained liquor. I don a pair of gloves and do a vaginal examination, but can feel nothing in the pelvis. She has a transverse lie, with her baby's head sitting over in the left iliac fossa. At least there is no cord prolapse and the foetal heart rate is strong and steady. I write a note for Andre and give it to Maheswary to take to him in theatre: 'Sending you an emergency Caesar!'

The rickety old trolley arrives and away she goes. Our cheerful orderly, Nedesh, expertly weaves the trolley through the crowded ward, between the beds, dodging mothers and babies lying on the floor. There's not enough beds for them all and anyway, it's cooler on the concrete.

The day progresses. A couple of births, some Depo injections. It's midday and the sweat is pouring off me in the immense heat. Indira, who had the incomplete miscarriage this morning, has returned from her D&C and is emerging from her ketamine-induced anaesthetic. She lies there half-crying, half-laughing and her bystander fans her with a piece of cardboard from the side of a powdered milk box. Ketamine is a safe anaesthetic, but it causes intense hallucinations as patients are waking. Mathilda, who had been sent off for the emergency

Caesarean section, is safe and her baby is well although a murky green colour from meconium. He needed some oxygen and suction at birth, but under the determined ministrations of our little volunteer hospital workers, he finally consents to breathe and join the human race! He lies beside his mother, blinking myopically into the light and feeling his grubby streaked face with tiny wrinkled fingers. His breathing is a little rattly, but he remains well-oxygenated. His grandmother hovers close by, ready to take him and wash him under the garden tap outside as soon as she can lay her hands on him.

Meanwhile the young woman with the dead baby is in labour. She writhes and moans and, as the day progresses, her wails become more urgent.

'*Indiamma, amoy, Indiamma*,' she cries, calling for her mother. I keep a close eye on her, looking for any sign of imminent rupture. There is no pain relief available here, so labour must be endured in all its terrible splendour. A box of glucose powder is the most important thing to pack when coming to hospital to give birth. The bystander pours it into her cupped hand and tips it into the mouth of the sweating mother, helping her to wash it down with some tepid water from the old Fanta bottle every woman keeps beside her.

Suddenly the woman with the APH begins to bleed again. Clots everywhere, foetal heart okay. 'Andre – guess what?' Off she goes for an emergency Caesarean. Out comes another shocked little Tamil, loath to breathe but finally signing on for the ride. By now the place is starting to look decidedly war-torn. Bodies, babies, bystanders, IV poles, flies, heat, bottles of water, women labouring and moaning.

The mother with her dead baby is pushing. She bears down valiantly and the mauve scalp becomes visible. We stand with her, urging her on to greater efforts. But there is no progress. Over the next two hours the contractions begin to fade, becoming slower and weaker. She is exhausted, drifting out of labour and needs more oxytocin to stimulate her. Time goes by, and my anxiety rises. What is happening to her uterus? I daren't stimulate it further in case she ruptures, but she must be delivered. We can't wait much longer. I speak with Andre and he decides to take her to theatre to deliver her there, probably by doing a foetal destruction. He has never done one before and has his emergency obstetrics procedure book out skimming the diagrams. It is now 5 pm. The little boy is finally born after some grisly manoeuvres to enable him to slip out. The grief-stricken family is waiting anxiously for their beloved daughter and wife to return safely to them. I carry her baby boy back to the labour room. He is perfect in every way. I wash him and wrap him so that his injured head is covered, then gently pass him to his father who breaks into wrenching sobs as he cradles his second dead son. I turn away and break down myself. It all seems so unfair. They weren't asking for too much, were they? Just a healthy child. The Hindu religion stipulates that he must be buried before the sun sets, so they take him away to his final resting place. At the same time I am summoned to theatre to try and remove the adherent placenta. It won't separate and I have to don a glove and attempt my first manual removal. A very weird sensation and I keep in mind the possibility of pushing my finger through her uterine scar. It's scary.

The woman with the hypertension is now fully dilated and pushing. Her baby's head is on view and there is lots of moulding. It's nearly 7 pm. I ask Karmela to call me when she is ready for delivery. I go to the compound for my first break for the day to have a meal but am not hungry. There is too much to think about. Nine o'clock comes and no call. I set off again into the night, carrying the torch and holding the two-way radio. No further progress. Darling Karmela is still there, looking worried and weary. I try every trick I know in the book. Standing, squatting, rocking, fundal pressure. Nothing happens. I feel way out of my depth here. I can't do a forceps, or a ventouse, and nor can anyone else here. My heart rate is up. I'm very anxious.

Suddenly I remember something a trusted friend told me before I left Australia: 'Everything you need is inside you.' It steadies me. After another hour of pushing, shoving, praying and swearing (silently), I finally say to Andre: 'This isn't going to happen. Fancy another Caesarean?'

'Shit,' he says. 'How will I get the head out? You'll have to come in and push it up from the vagina.' Another steep learning curve about to happen.

The generator starts up and lights come on. We scrub, Marina injects the ketamine, Andre cuts. The glistening swollen uterus bulges forward. He cuts, clamps, ties off, cuts again.

'Suction!'

The ancient sucker gurgles into life, sipping the amniotic fluid away as it flows out of her wound. There is the baby! All mauve and squash-faced, lying on his back, face upwards. A posterior position with a deflexed head – no wonder we couldn't budge him!

'Okay push his head up now,' says Andre urgently, as his hand delves deep into her uterus trying to release the impacted head. We are both dripping sweat. I crouch on the floor under the ragged drapes, and slip my hand into her vagina. I feel Andre's fingers coming down from inside and our fingertips touch briefly. I push the baby's head and it floats up out of the pelvis like an egg slipping out of an egg-cup. She has a son! The umbilical cord is clamped and cut and his flaccid body is passed to Marina for resuscitation. He is alive, stunned and huge. Some oxygen, some suction, some vigorous rubbing and he begins to cry. Thank God – he's okay. This means large amounts of sugar crystals will be handed around to all and sundry over the next few days. Soft wrapped lollies for girl babies and lumps of sugar crystals for boys.

I finally walk home at 11.30 pm after a day I don't care to repeat. Jane and Agnetha have waited up for me. What a joy to walk into the compound and see the welcome glow of the kerosene lamps and be welcomed by my friends. I sink into a hammock, drain another cold bottle of soda water and we talk quietly for a while. It is over, they are safe, there is a bright moon shining and no sounds of shelling in the distance. Just me, the girls, the guards, and some feral dogs fighting down the lane.

So, what did I learn that day? That everything I needed I really did have – both within me and beside me. Our expat team, Karmela our wonderful midwife, our brave mothers and their families. The oxygen of friendship and teamwork, where to have support and encouragement is life-sustaining. Second, that you don't need much to do good. Decision-making in this environment is easy, because the choices are so few and so stark.

Do nothing and they die, do something and a life may be saved. The 'something' was also pretty basic. No machines to dictate our clinical responses. It all came back to very fundamental surgical and midwifery skills.

Finally, the resilience and courage of these women, who walk with death and cope with what life hands them every time they give birth, was a humbling experience for me.

Just another day? No way.

On the road with Infant Welfare

OLIVIA LANGLEY

I've always loved working with children, so it was a natural career move to go into Infant Welfare, as it was called back in 1963. I had a position in charge of the Mount Barker Infant Welfare Centre, 350 kilometres south of Perth. This was my main centre. Once a week I would hold a clinic at Denmark, and fortnightly I would go to Cranbrook and other small towns. In the clinics we still wore a uniform and a large white veil on our head. For home and hospital visits we dispensed with the veil, which was more relaxing for everyone.

Today is a Thursday, and I'm off to visit an Aboriginal camp. It's a good hour's drive to reach my destination. The main road is a smooth one and there are frequent lines of gum trees along its sides. I sing to pass the time. There is no tape deck or CD player in the car, so it's just my voice. Gilbert and Sullivan songs are my current favourites.

At last I reach the turn-off. The road is rougher now – bump . . . bump . . . bump. I turn into a clearing where there are a few old canvas tents and shanties. Outside one I see three Aboriginal boys playing with stones, seeing how far they can throw them. My window is open and I can hear the little song one of them is singing:

Ah there nigger boong nigger boong nigger boong,
Ah there nigger boong . . .

and so on. These boys are not even school age but they must have been taunted and they know they are different from the other boys in the town. I wave to them, and they turn to look at the car and who's inside it. I drive to the end of the roadway and park.

Now I open the boot and uncover my scales. A large, shapeless Aboriginal woman comes out of a tent and strolls up.

'Hello!' I say. 'I just want to weigh the babies. Is Sally Dodds there?'

'Yeah, she's just coming. There's her an' Flo. Be there in a minute.'

I wait, and wait. Meanwhile, a semicircle of small boys and girls are gathering around the back of the car, to see the fun. A scrawny brown kitten appears and jumps into the boot. I put him out again as fast as he got in.

At last the two mothers, Sally and Flo, appear out of the tent in front of us. Sally tells me that her baby's name is Bull-bull. Flo's is to be called Smiley. The babies are dressed in clean shirts and snow-white towelling nappies. Later I learn that the nappies were put on just for my visit, which explains the wait. Whatever the babies normally wear or don't wear, it's a fact that I've never seen a sore bottom at the Aboriginal camp, but I see plenty at the clinics frequented by their fairer sisters and brothers.

As I'm weighing Smiley I feel a light tingle on my leg – a beetle, perhaps? I look down and there is a small dark boy touching my leg.

'Sorry about that, Sis!' says his mother, pulling him away. 'You see, he's never seen no one with stockings on before.'

Another day I am visiting Flo and Bull-bull, who is now one month old. I weigh the baby and enter the details on his card.

'And how often do you feed him?' I ask, intending to record 'three-' or 'four-hourly.' Flo looks at me as if I'm silly. 'When he's hungry!' she replies.

So, who is the one with common sense? Some months later I'm speaking to a senior nurse in Perth and recounting this tale. She smiles and comments: 'You never need to tell an Aboriginal mother how to breastfeed a baby. They know more than we'll ever know.'

On another visit, the baby Smiley has bad conjunctivitis, what we called a 'sticky eye'.

'You'd better see the doctor about that one,' I say.

A fortnight later I'm back to weigh the babies again. Smiley's eye is clear and bright, and I comment on how good it looks.

'So, you saw the doctor?' I ask.

'Nuh,' said the mother. 'I fixed it our way.'

'Oh. And what do you do?'

'I put some breast milk in it!'

Since then, when I see a baby with conjunctivitis, I suggest to a breastfeeding mother that, as well as bathing the eye, she treat it with a squirt of breast milk now and then. It works!

In another country town where I have an afternoon clinic, I'm told of a sick baby at the Aboriginal camp. I call in there and a worried mother shows me into her tent. Lying on some old blankets on the ground is a little fellow called Bob, about nine months old. His eyes are dull; he looks listless and is off his food. I offer to take him back with me to the hospital at Mount Barker, and the mother agrees. I settle him as safely as I can on the floor in the back of the car, for there are no seat belts. Carefully I drive back the 100 kilometres to Mount Barker and the hospital. Matron Turner is on duty, so I explain the position to her, and hand young Bob over to her care. He is placed in a comfortable cot, fed and seen by the doctor on his next visit.

Over the next ten days his medical condition is treated and his health improves. Then suddenly, he dies.

I often wonder about that baby. What a culture shock it must have been for him to be taken from his warm black mother and his bed of blankets among his brothers and sisters. Then to be driven away and put in a white sheeted cot with white bars around it and tended by pale women in starched uniforms. I wonder would it have made any difference to the outcome, had I called in after work each day to nurse the child and talk to him. Looking back over the years I can see that I should have taken his mother, too. It would have been difficult for her to stay at the hospital, but I may have been able to help.

Infant welfare nursing is isolating work and can be lonely. When problems arise, one misses having other nurses to confer with.

At one clinic I had a new pair of portable scales, which were useful when visiting a baby at home for the first visit. After work, I packed these scales into the boot of the car and went to visit a new mother, Mrs Lynda Taylor, and her baby who lived in a flat behind the general store where her husband worked. The baby was called Maxine, and she was doing well. Mrs Taylor undressed Maxine ready for weighing and I took the cover off the scales. It was only then that I discovered that a vital piece of the scales was missing. I was very apologetic. The grandmother, who was watching, had a good idea.

'I wonder,' she said. 'The post office scales?'

We all trooped into the back door of the post office. Maxine's grandmother worked there, so she had the key. Fortunately it was after-hours, so there were no customers. I carefully balanced the bare baby on the scales used for small parcels. This baby was indeed a 'small parcel', so she just fitted and two pairs of hands were ready in case she gave a sudden kick. I made a quick check of the dial below the scales, and handed her back to her mother, to have the nappy replaced.

Those scales must have weighed many a Christmas present, but none as precious as this one.

Broken waters

SUSAN TIMPANI

I love the flight out of Sydney at dusk. The plane climbs over the lights of the city, skirts the majestic Opera House and Harbour Bridge and leaves behind the brilliant orange sky over the Quay. On my last trip, I left Australia as a graduate midwife from Sydney Maternity Hospital. After a number of flight changes, with each plane getting smaller, I finally found myself trekking under the awesome canopy of the Papua New Guinea jungle.

In single file, our group moved quickly through the mosquito-infested trail. My lilywhite legs attracted the mozzies like moths to a light bulb and the resulting bites drove me nearly insane. I looked behind at Tersia, my teenage patient, to encourage her to keep pace. Tersia had grown up sure-footed in this soggy tangle of roots.

However, hacking through it during the 38th week of her twin pregnancy was proving to be a different and significant challenge for her.

Over his shoulder, Papiali aimed a tirade of local words at his struggling wife. He waved his arms and pointed above the solid trees. Tersia lowered her eyes and, true to custom, gave no reply.

'Here, take my hand!' I stretched back my arm and clutched Tersia's wrist.

I shook off droplets of rain that trickled from yellow-green palm leaves on to my loose curls. Feeling uneasy, my eyes scanned the rainforest. Among the myriad tropical plants, resplendent birds sang, each with its own song. I inhaled the paradisiacal wonder and knew that I would carry this privilege with me always. Just as I would re-live the irony. It was imperative that we move quickly.

'*Mi no gat strong*. I'm not strong enough.' Tersia's frightened whisper could be heard as she gasped for breath in the heavy air.

'You're doing really well.' I held back a smile at my absurd words. My instinctive labour ward response didn't quite have the same punch as it had back in Sydney.

But what else could I tell her? Tersia's young, lightly tattooed face looked up at me. Her dark eyes were defenceless against nature.

My own eyes were panicky. Over the past three hours I had watched her cumbersome pregnant load sap her strength. Every breath was audible due to the combination of severe anaemia and extreme humidity.

Tightening my grip on Tersia's emaciated arm, I exhorted: '*Liklik tasol*. Just a little longer.' A tiny grin broke the tension around her lips. *Liklik* was an ambiguous term. We both knew it could mean a few minutes or a few hours.

I was the only registered midwife between this trackless jungle and the hospital, the latter accessible only by light aircraft. Our dirt airstrip back in Blonga had to be dry for the plane to land. From the moment I examined Tersia in her village of Uti, selecting the best option for her care weighed in my mind like a pendulum.

Our group had stayed in Uti for a few days for my maternal and child health clinic. On the last morning, while packing away the gear from the outdoor clinic, Tersia caught my eye. Hardly more than a child herself, I thought: how will she manage pregnancy, birth and parenting? I unhooked the scales from the tree and removed the attached baby hammock. I stored in the metal tin the glass syringes and stainless steel needles used for the immunisations. They would be sterilised in a strong alcohol solution when I arrived back in Blonga later that afternoon.

I gently tapped Tersia's shoulder, as she sat among a group of women. 'Can I check your tummy?'

Her shy smile indicated assent and a couple of women hoisted her up, leading us into a thatched hut on stilts. The perpetual sizzle of charcoal permeated the single room with smoke. One of the women picked up a bundle of sticks tied with rope and swept a clean space for us on the floor. Adjusting my eyes to the dimness of the room, I gently opened Tersia's laplap, her wrap-around dress. It was impossible not to feel self-conscious as the women settled into a circle to watch. However, their chatter and laughter faded into an inaudible backdrop as I faced the challenging results of my check.

It was the same nerve-racking findings each time I repeated the examination. My fingers crept across Tersia's full-term uterus again. Tucked just beneath her rib cage lay a rock-hard mass, while another hovered above the brim of her pelvis. Pushing aside my fearful questions, I took out the stethoscope and calmly continued examining her.

True to nurse training, my face contained all my insecurity behind its confident mask. With a smile I announced, '*Tupela*.' Tersia was having twins. The phrase: 'One of the twins is in the breech position,' went beyond my Pidgin vocabulary. A lot of giggles followed my attempt to mime instead.

Absently, I took Tersia's arm and helped her to sit up, leaned back on my haunches and considered the options. The women usually helped each other to deliver, calling on the aid post midwife only if there was complications. This patient required even more care than I could offer from a simple aid post.

'Tersia, you need the *haus sik*, the hospital.' The women's chatter ceased, mouths chewing betel nut clamped shut and Tersia buried her face into her chest. Then the storm of words began. They gabbled to each other, to Tersia, to me, and eventually a message was even sent to the men outside. Was it such a preposterous suggestion?

I mentally checked through the list. Tersia was a teenager in her first pregnancy. She was having twins. At term, one baby was in the breech position and one had its head high above the brim of the pelvis. Even by PNG's standards, both babies were small for dates. Tersia's blood pressure was high; her haemoglobin registered low on the capillary meter, indicating probable anaemia. Her skinny frame bordered on malnutrition.

Tersia laid her hands lightly on top of mine and explained the chaos: '*Bikpela Wara*. The Big Rain.'

When I stepped outside, our trek leader, Kaki, translated the community's concerns from dialect into basic English. 'The Wet Season is now. Before long these showers will become the Big Rain and stay for many weeks.'

Tersia stood on the top step while Kaki continued: 'If we come safely through the jungle before the Big Rain' – he looked over at Tersia – 'and the babies don't come, we still must cross the river.'

On our way to Uti, the wide river was already high and rapid, but the timber swing bridge easily cleared it. There was just one more problem. If it rained too heavily, the muddy airstrip in Blonga could be closed for weeks. We had to leave soon, before that happened. 'It will be unsafe for me to come back here to help with Tersia's delivery. The *haus sik* is the safest place.'

Papiali, Tersia's husband, stepped forward and spat out his betel nut. His huge smile revealed a mouthful of red-stained teeth. Indicating the jungle ahead, he flung his arm flippantly, stating, '*Yu mi go*. We're going.'

I suspected that the plane ride to the mysterious world beyond the mountains was his motivation. Kaki nodded his agreement to move on. Trusting his experience, Tersia joined the team and we set out.

When we finally made it through the jungle, the river was terrifying. We stood watching the rapid, foaming force; its banks swollen to capacity. Branches from windswept trees rushed past, pushed along by the rapid current. There was no sign of the swing bridge to help us across.

Tersia and I sat on the ground with our arms around each other, too stunned to talk. Unable to hear above the noise, Kaki and Papiali gestured their discussion. Kaki came close to us and crouched down. His voice barely audible above the deafening roar, he urged: 'We must cross. Before long this bank will break and we'll be here for many weeks.'

'You must be mad!' I screamed to myself. I had never been so petrified in my life. Amazingly, Tersia gripped my shivering hand to reassure me. I had to trust the local people. They were survivors, not unnecessary risk-takers.

Obediently, we stepped into the cool, surging water, forming a human chain with Tersia and me in the middle, Kaki and Papiali on either side and a carrier at either end. My heart was thumping crazily as we waded across.

The water grew deeper and deeper until it swirled around my neck. I am short and the insipid foam splashed my tongue and lips. To clear the surface I had to tilt my head right back; the water just missed my ears.

Right in the middle of the river I felt Tersia lose her balance and pull me down. 'Kaki! Papiali!'

The men almost pulled our arms out of our sockets, but they managed to shove us upright again. Both of us women used every ounce of our strength and determination to keep our balance. I kept my eyes on the opposite bank and repeatedly told myself we were going to make it. We finally clambered up the embankment, thoroughly drenched, but safe. One of the carriers then went on ahead to arrange the plane.

Tersia and I lagged way behind the men. We walked in silence, but in my heart I told her: 'Just one more hour, Tersia, and you'll be safe.'

I didn't even know if they were tears that trickled along my nose, down my cheeks and into my mouth. The sticky, sultry wet of the atmosphere and the river all blended into one. I was so weary. 'Just one more hour, Susan,' I told myself, 'and you can call it a day.'

Suddenly, Tersia's face came to life. Grabbing my hand, she dragged me along. Signalling the sky, she cried, '*Balus! Balus!* The plane! The plane!'

We arrived at Blonga to see the single-engine Cessna come into view. The villagers gathered along the sides of the airstrip to watch this great event. The plane thundered as it descended and finally landed. When the pilot emerged, I had never been so happy to hear an Aussie voice.

'G'day!' he smiled, and tossed me a much-awaited mailbag.

After a brief discussion all around, Tersia and I hugged each other. '*Tenkyu, tenkyu tru.*'

'Thank you, thank you so much,' I replied, and we parted.

As the plane disappeared over the mountains, I realised that during the whole expedition Tersia hadn't shown any signs of being in labour.

Eight weeks later, following the Big Rain, Tersia and Papiali returned with their tiny healthy twins. Twin One was named after Dad: Papiali. Twin Two was called Susan.

The people of perpetual spring

MARIE TRELOAR

Our land is the island of high mountains,
Of sunlit palms and coral sea,
Where our people sing while the drums are beating,
For our land is strong and free,
Papua . . . New Guinea . . .
(G. Baskett, song, 'Papua New Guinea')

A four-hour journey by aeroplane takes me to a nation of perpetual spring, where the people's smiles are brighter than the prospects of surviving past the age of 50. A people with a sense of eternal peace despite the lack of material possessions and a life that offers little hope for recovery if sickness or pain comes their way. A community called Goroka is my destination.

Goroka is a major commercial centre of 25,000 people in the Eastern Highlands of Papua New Guinea (PNG). It has a history of gold mines and coffee plantations and a temperate sunny climate.

Why do I go? I want to volunteer my midwifery skills and knowledge to help a culture less socially and economically fortunate than our own. I want to be influenced by another culture and other ways of coping with birth and health complications. I want to experience a different healthcare system and to see how women birth outside the obstetrical dominance of the Western world. I want to discover the beauty, traditions and uniqueness of a country like PNG.

How do we make it happen? A local obstetrician/gynaecologist, Dr Ian Hoffman (fondly known as Hoffy), spent some time as a young resident living and working in PNG. He is now retired from private practice but dedicates his time to travelling to Goroka three times a year to work as an O&G consultant. With a love for the people, he has been drawn back to this beautiful country, giving his operative skills and knowledge, using his own resources. On his recommendation, I have now been to PNG twice and hope to return regularly to continue this labour of love, which began as an adventure and has developed into a quest to help improve the health of the beautiful and uncomplaining people of PNG.

My first trip was in 2003. General Nurse Nadia Ellery and midwifery student Nicole Tydall decided to join me on this three-week working holiday. The team was established, and after making contact with the director of nursing at the Goroka Base Hospital and gaining approval for our visit, we registered with the Nursing

Council of PNG. Once we had negotiated the necessary passports, visas and letters of approval we applied for annual leave and set off on a life-changing adventure.

In Port Moresby, the humidity and heat took our breath away. A small Fokker aeroplane waited to take us to Goroka and, for the final leg of the journey, the hospital's rickety old four-wheel-drive jeep (which doubled as the ambulance), took us to Mendekwe Lodge, a local guesthouse. This was a secure building with high mesh fences and 24-hour armed security gatekeepers. Visitors are expected to reside this way in PNG. Safety is a major issue, and law and order is a top priority for the PNG government as it endeavours to stabilise the nation. Unfortunately, the negative incidents with 'rascals' and expatriates portrayed in the media have given PNG a reputation of being an unsafe place to visit, work and live. With this knowledge we kept ourselves out of vulnerable situations and befriended the community and felt safe at all times. Goroka's remoteness, in fact, makes it one of the safest places in PNG, and incidents are more common in the coastal areas.

As in many places in the world, violence against women is a serious issue. Cultural ways and lack of family planning give rise to high birth rates which, in turn, contribute to dangerously high infant and maternal mortality rates.

We stayed in a very dilapidated two-bedroom unit with only bare essentials in the kitchen, not even hotplates. However, we were grateful for this clean and safe place which was to become our home for the next three weeks. As we tried to open tins with knives and to toast our bread on the stove elements, we began to miss the luxuries of home. However, as the days passed the items we so craved appeared with the compliments of hotel management.

We made the most of the remaining daylight on our first day by going into the town centre to buy food at the local supermarket. Every eye was upon us as we searched for new brands and different foods. These curious faces were soon to become familiar faces who would say *good monin* and *apenun* to us whenever we walked the streets of Goroka to the open-air markets, hospital or town centre.

On our first official morning, we dressed in our work outfits and headed off to the hospital where we were greeted by the director of nursing who took us on a comprehensive tour and introduced us to the staff. We tried to learn and remember the names of the many friendly and welcoming staff of this *haus sick* (hospital) who were to become like family over the next few weeks.

We were given the rest of the day off and so we walked back into town to see the many handmade items for sale, such as the *bilims* (crocheted bags), which are unique to this nation. Every Papuan owns a *bilim* – it's used to carry everything from newborn babies to fruit and vegetables, Bibles and other personal belongings. I now have a stunning collection of about twenty bilims, given to me as gifts from new friends made while in this beautiful country.

On our first day at work, Nicole and I found our way to the labour ward. The ward was empty, so we spent the day working in the special care baby nursery. There were nine babies there, ranging in weight from 1.19 to 3.3 kilograms. Most were underweight premature babies with compromising conditions ranging from neonatal sepsis and pneumonia to congenital syphilis and tetanus. We didn't know how premature these babies were, as the mothers usually didn't know their dates and ultrasound was only available for those who could afford it.

It was poignant to see the mothers come in at feed times and sit on the floor and hand-express enough breast milk for the feeds. They would then cup-feed those babies who were able to tolerate this method of feeding, and we tube-fed the breast milk to those babies who couldn't suck or swallow well. I truly believe that the expressed breast milk was a major factor in keeping these babies alive, considering the poor conditions of the nursery and the lack of resources to provide intensive care for them.

However, the loss of babies was never easy to accept. When we came back from morning tea on that first day, we heard the tragic news of baby Joe's death. Joe was 3.3 kilograms and had suffered from neonatal sepsis and tetanus. He had arrested the previous day. The nurses had attempted resuscitation by suctioning and frog breathing, with no success. Given the lack of response, the doctors didn't feel they could do anything more. There was no ventilator or tracheotomy tubes to perform any advanced resuscitation. Indeed, there is no option of flying to Port Moresby for advanced care unless parents or patients have money.

Baby Joe's mother was called from the ward and told of his death. After a short time of grief, she was expected to take him to her village and prepare him for burial. The cot was cleaned and we moved on.

The staff at Goroka Hospital estimate that they lose one baby every fortnight. The reality of their desperate situation was again highlighted as we tried to help another baby survive, whose oxygen saturations were 59–65 per cent. We couldn't find appropriate suction catheters. We improvised by cutting tubes and putting them inside others to make the suction work. This, however, wasn't the only difficulty. All available oxygen was used up overnight, so we had to wait for the next supply to arrive from the larger city of Lae. We did manage to stabilise the baby on oxygen saturation of 99 per cent, but sadly the little one died overnight. The acceptance of life and death by the native people was amazing. We too began to accept it and do what we could, never expecting too much.

After spending a few days in the special care nursery, we decided it was time to experience the labour ward. Margaret was the first woman in our care. She was 8 centimetres dilated on arrival. Someone brought her from the village and then left her to labour alone. It was sweltering outside and Margaret was told to have a cold shower before going to her bed in the open birthing suite. Surrounded by seven beds partitioned by not-so-private curtains, she laboured silently. We assisted Margaret by massaging her back and supporting her. This type of midwife care, where midwives actually stay with the woman, was foreign to the nurses/midwives who worked in the labour ward. Most of the staff were general nurses skilled in birth suite. They were multiskilled: attending the women's episiotomies, perineal suturing, ventouse extractions and IV cannulations.

Nicole assisted Margaret in her normal vaginal birth. She had a lovely 3.6-kilogram baby boy. I received the baby and administered the routine care of suctioning, weighing, measuring, administering Hepatitis B vaccine, vitamin K, polio sabine syrup and chloromycetin eye ointment.

During labour, massage and movement are the only forms of pain relief available. The resuscitation cot was archaic; a wooden trolley with a light, no heat and a hard plastic tray. The suction and oxygen available is by portable means only. The same suction machine used for ventouse extractions is then used for suctioning babies' airways. After rinsing in water between births, the same suction catheter was used for all the babies.

After the babies are born they are wrapped in a thin muslin wrap brought in by the mothers, as well as any other wraps they have. The cot has a plastic mattress. If the mother isn't interested in holding her baby, midwives do it to help retain warmth. The mother is then expected to get her things together, have another cold shower and transfer to the postnatal ward. We naturally couldn't stop ourselves from helping these women, who seemed to be doing it quite tough.

We were to have many beautiful and natural births during our three-week stay. Thrown in were the occasional postpartum haemorrhages requiring four to six units of blood, undiagnosed FDIUs (foetal deaths in utero) and twin births. We were touched to hear that one of the mothers we had helped to recover from a postpartum haemorrhage named her twin girls Nicole and Marie.

Our style of woman-centred care was well received by the nurses/midwives, who acknowledged the need to practise in a similar way. Women didn't get pampered as they do in the West. They were expected to get on with the process of labour and birth in a natural way, hence there were many normal births with minimal intervention. We were amazed at the power of the women, and by their strength and courage. They never asked for anything and were grateful for any small act of kindness. We felt drawn to help these women as much as we could and to make them feel worthy.

My experience in the labour ward area was memorable and filled with joy. However, I spent quite a lot of time teaching and advising the staff and students in the medical, special care nursery, paediatric and labour wards. As I worked with them, I was able to instruct them in areas where they lacked skills and knowledge, such as physiotherapy, care of the unconscious patient, general nursing care, lifting techniques and neonatal resuscitation. It was very rewarding to see changes take place soon after they had been suggested. I was also able to gather together nurse unit managers and supervisors who were eager to receive education on time management, teamwork, staff efficiency, prioritising care, basic nursing care, health education for patients and relatives, collaboration, code of conduct, indemnity issues, and practising within their nursing responsibilities.

The nurses were concerned that they were expected to do too many medical procedures. They had been accustomed, for too long, to the lack of medical staff. The nurses expressed a sense of powerlessness, yet understood that a unified effort was needed to change the culture that centred on medical procedures and neglected nursing care.

My short time in Goroka was very rewarding. The positive feedback received from the staff and people proved that we had made a difference. The staff sent a message home with me to share with everyone in Australia – they hoped that more Australian nurses and midwives would travel to Goroka and experience this warm and friendly town and hospital.

The nurses and midwives in Goroka would also appreciate the opportunity to experience work and life in Australia. Unfortunately, lack of finances makes such opportunities rare. I believe that because we have so much, it is our responsibility to share with our neighbours all that we can. I have been touched and moved to take an active part in helping the people of Goroka.

A lot has been achieved since my first visit to the town. Together with Hoffy, Dr David Laurie and his daughter Kate Laurie, we have been able to establish The Highlands Foundation, which is committed to improving the health of women, children and their families in the Highlands of PNG.

Something wonderful is happening here. We have been able to coordinate regular teams of doctors, nurses and midwives to go to Goroka on short-term trips to provide help where needed. The generosity of the Australian people has enabled us to pack a shipping container with necessary hospital, medical and baby supplies, and funds raised by Rotary clubs have met the shipping costs.

We have also been able to organise sponsorship for three nurses/midwives from Goroka to visit Australia for conferences and professional experiences to empower them to help their community.

Although The Highlands Foundation has been formed by Australians, we have already received support internationally from developed countries and plan to continue this work.

This is only one example of how midwives and health professionals can share their skills, knowledge and resources to help make a difference for people in developing countries who, unlike us in the West, struggle to achieve even a basic level of health and quality of life.

Find out more about The Highlands Foundation at www.highlandsfoundation.org.au

It's an airborne knockout!

JUDY THOMSON

Do we ever stop to think of the impact that midwives and doctors have on the lives of childbearing women?

Back in the late 1980s I was working in women's health and was fortunate to be a part of many memorable maternity cases. Take, for example, the case of Thelma, an Aboriginal woman born and bred in Wilcannia, a historic river town on the Darling River in far western New South Wales. Wilcannia formed an important transport hub that helped open up the area. The river united communities along its path.

Nowadays the paddle-steamers are gone, but the Darling River continues to snake its way through the dry and unforgiving countryside surrounding Wilcannia. This is the special land of the Barkengee people. Grey-blue saltbush dots the red earth, which is a wonderful contrast to the brightest of bright blue skies. The vastness is amazing, particularly if you come from a busy metropolitan region. The stillness in the air and the constant cry of crows evokes a spiritual sense. The remoteness of such places actually cocoons them and makes them special to visit. It was a privilege to work there.

Thelma had six children aged from one to ten years. She was 27 years old and her priority was to care for all her kids. Her partner, Steve, was often away from home looking for work on outback stations. She was now heavily pregnant with her seventh child and was due to deliver soon.

The population of Wilcannia was at the time less than 1000. It was a predominantly Aboriginal community with a small bush hospital. This health facility only had a few beds and no blood bank, so it was decreed that births would take place at the nearest large hospital, in Broken Hill, over 200 kilometres away.

The need for evacuation was difficult to explain to clients and their families. It is still commonplace in remote areas such as Wilcannia, due to the lack of staff and appropriate resources. It's difficult to advocate for your clients when you are also aware of the many risk factors involved in not evacuating. It's a perennial problem – weighing up the social isolation and disruption suffered by families against pressing health and safety needs.

It's also very difficult to translate 'Western' medical rules to people who are closely bonded to their children and extended families. Why should they be required to leave their home environments for something that is supposed to be as natural as childbirth? Imagine being taken out of your own surroundings, accompanied by strangers, put on a small aircraft (even more alarming if you have never flown before) – add to that taking off, flying and then landing in an unfamiliar place – then a trip in an ambulance for several kilometres to a large town hospital. Upon arrival at the hospital the woman is transferred to the maternity section with its large clinical labour wards that definitely don't smell like home.

The women of Wilcannia naturally shared their birthing experiences and tried to avoid such trips.

Thelma wanted her seventh child to be born in Wilcannia, with no separation from her children or her family. Less disruption all round. She almost pulled it off, too.

She was at the Royal Flying Doctor Service (RFDS) clinic being treated for a chest infection and started to have labour pains while there, which you may say was not good timing on her part. The doctor was adamant that she must be transferred to deliver her baby in Broken Hill.

Thelma protested, but to no avail. She told the doctor that her baby would 'come real soon', but he continued with the paperwork. Thelma wasn't impressed – she was, after all, only having a baby. Surely all this intervention was unnecessary? I felt torn between the two options, as I was well aware of how much Thelma wanted to remain at home. I was also aware that as this was her seventh baby there was an increased risk of postpartum haemorrhage, and with no blood bank facilities we would be taking a huge risk not to evacuate her.

Perhaps with knowledge came fear.

Although this doctor was new to the bush and to the RFDS he did, of course, know best. Admittedly, I thought he was handsome, with a wonderful smile, and he was well aware of his good looks. He almost looked the part, too, in his yet to be worn-in moleskins and new R.M. Williams boots. I don't think he was game to add an Akubra hat. That would have been overkill. As he was new to medical practice in the outback, his need for reassurance far outweighed that of Thelma, who really knew her stuff.

The pilot had only just taken off when Thelma's labour began in earnest.

I knew it wouldn't be long and, sure enough, she suddenly changed dramatically from a quiet, subdued woman to one who seemed possessed. The doctor had also only completed the absolute minimum obstetrical training requirements at the time, so he found the yelling and bellowing overwhelming, to say the least. Working space was limited inside the small aircraft. He tried to reason with Thelma but she was, understandably, not in a receptive mood. I was seated across the aisle from her and she gripped my hand incessantly. There was little time and space for me to do more.

With a final blood-curdling yell from Thelma, the baby literally flew through the air. I managed to grab the little thing who, thankfully, was fine. As the shocked doctor attempted to give the mother an injection to help with expulsion of the placenta, she accidentally knocked him to one side of the plane. He hit the floor and remained motionless for a second or two. The syringe was somewhere down on the floor – not to be located until the plane was being cleaned after the event.

The mother was feeling good – she was now grinning at the doctor and me – triumphant. Drama over. She had given birth to a healthy little boy and we hadn't flown far out of Wilcannia. The doctor was now back in his seat rubbing his chin where Thelma's fist had connected. But once the aircraft had left Wilcannia it was bound for Broken Hill. Thelma needed to be fully assessed at the base hospital in Broken Hill, so there was no turnaround.

We were absolutely covered in body fluids. (Thank goodness, we had no blood rule then.) I hardly dared glance at the new young doctor – he seemed so shocked by the events. His lovely beige moleskins were covered in blood and gunk. It had been some knockout!

The next day I went to visit Thelma and her little boy in hospital in Broken Hill. She laughed at the act she had put on – she even asked how the doctor was now. I suggested to her that she should name her boy after him, and she laughed and winked at me.

I'd lay a bet that the memory of that birthing experience is one that makes that doctor squirm a little even today. He's a highly regarded leading specialist now . . . but not in obstetrics.

On the train line

PRUE O'HALLORAN

I left for Western Australia in the mid-1980s with a friend. So confident of passing our midwifery exams, we were in Perth by the time we got the results. After talking to another midwifery student we chose Kalgoorlie – or Kal, as we later called it – for our outback adventure.

We were in our mid-twenties and were totally unprepared for the challenge that lay ahead. We knew nothing of Aboriginal culture, let alone how to nurse Aboriginal people. We were Sydneysiders. I hailed from near Bondi Beach. Crashing waves coupled with beautiful headlands and rock pools would now be replaced by red dust – lots of it. Two decades later, the sight of red dust still heals the very essence of my soul when it feels depleted.

The old weatherboard nurses' home at Kalgoorlie Regional Hospital (or KRH, as it was known) became home to Australian, Irish and English girls who were all in the same boat as us visitors to this big state. We brought universal nursing skills and experience, caring, youthful exuberance, vitality, laughter, and an eagerness to have fun and to learn.

We were naïve, but we were fortunate to work with many wise bush nurses while there.

We didn't dare think past six months. Well, that's what we told all our Sydney friends.

We stayed for over three years. Matron was so proud of us and happily showed us off. New staff would be orientated when 'Prue and Sue' were on. Matron would introduce us and then say, 'Prue and Sue, how long have you been here now, girls?'

In our own way we also contributed to, and made a difference to, the fabric that made up KRH during our time there.

Before working as a midwife I was sent to Paediatrics. Nursing post-operative grommets and tonsillectomies was the sum total of my paediatric experience. I had much to learn. Paediatrics was a huge 45-bed ward, and these mostly Aboriginal kids were seriously ill. Every week the Royal Flying Doctor Service (RFDS) would evacuate kids with gastro, meningitis, and ear and chest infections from the communities in the Great Victoria Desert to our north, and along the 'Trans Line' to the east. There I learned to nurse small babies who barely cried, went limp in your arms as you held them, and had both sunken fontanelles and sunken eyes from dehydration. Their eyes were glazed over. The doctors couldn't get IVs into their shut-down veins, and every hour I would tenderly crane their little heads forward to give them oral electrolyte solution on a teaspoon. At times I could almost palpate their tenuous hold on life. Over time they would turn from fragile, limp rag dolls to babies with the biggest, brightest eyes that I had ever seen.

Nursing in the bush is often a sink-or-swim affair. On my first shift they put me into a four-bed isolation room for toddlers with gastro who were soon to be discharged. Not long after entering the room, I was stunned to see three-year-olds who simply pulled out their mother's breast whenever they wanted a drink. I had come from a place where we ruthlessly pursued the now archaic 'test weigh'. The procedure is thus: weigh babe with dry nappy, breastfeed, weigh babe with nappy and contents = feed taken. This was ideal in four-hourly regular feeds. Aboriginal children still on the breast can have very frequent feeds, and that day those children were in full swing. They had a lot of weight to catch up on. So I was weighing these children all day and doing my sums, just like they had taught me at my small Catholic midwifery hospital in Sydney's CBD.

'Better see what that new one's doing. We haven't seen her all day,' one of the nurses remarked, near the end of the shift. She found me immersed in arithmetic from calculations on every breastfeed those toddlers had during the shift. The paper spilled on to the floor and out the door – and what's more, I was proud of my maths.

'Oh, we don't do that here, love!'

They laughed about it for weeks.

Twenty years ago, pregnant women from remote areas stayed up to ten weeks in Kal, depending on complications. Of course they weren't all 'patients' unless there were problems, but they often chose to stay with us in Maternity, simply called Maty. Being in hospital meant actively staying away from the alcohol, found around the hostel in town. We looked after women from two different language groups and, as well as violence within the communities, there was also conflict between communities. They were brought to us by the RFDS, and most often this was their first time away from their desert communities, let alone travelling in a small plane. Teenage pregnancies were common, and we worked with their fears and uncertainties. I always felt privileged to be allowed into their world, a world so far removed from my own. I had to build trust with them, and it was a process of breaking down a void I didn't initially know how to cross.

The train line between the east and west of Australia ran past our back door.

That's where Aboriginal patients from KRH would gather. The men would light a fire, and a mob or two would sit out there all day. Once the women had their babies they would head to the train line, leaving the babies in our care for the day. Midwives would often be seen singing out loudly to the new mums to come and feed their babies. At dusk they would head home to Maty. We were home, while their real home was 1000 kilometres away in the desert. They got homesick. They missed other children. They felt confined in

Kal at times. But they knew it had to be. We became their family.

The women always bought their bras from the 'op shop'. A big group of our patients would head off there for the morning, replete with instructions from us on bra sizes. However, they would often buy a size 32A; when laden with milk, they had breasts pushed up under their chin. They didn't want a larger size, so we had to accept their decisions. Of course, they didn't wear bras in desert communities.

We shared so many intimate moments that still stay in my soul even after all these years. On one occasion I went into a four-bed room early in my afternoon shift.

Aboriginal girls are shy, and on this day they were giggling, whispering and being bashful in my presence. I was fascinated by the way they shrugged me off. This continued for a few hours until it dawned on another midwife that I had had my hair permed that day. They couldn't see that I was still Prue until I let them gently feel the tight curls that now adorned my head.

Most Aboriginal women I cared for laboured very quietly. They often just took to their bed and we might casually notice them as we walked past in our haste. An enquiry of 'baby pains?' usually gave us our answer with a nod. They had difficult labours at times and sick babies, but that wasn't the case with Bessie. This was to be her last baby and Bessie was to have a tubal ligation with her elective Caesarean section. Sterilisation required consent from both partners during my time there. Bessie's time with us had been both normal and routine. Her baby was born healthy and Bessie enjoyed the subsequent bonding time with her little one.

On the day Bessie was discharged, something strange happened. Aboriginal patients at KRH started absconding from the wards. It wasn't always easy to keep track of them during the day, especially those who sat out by the 'Trans Line'. Their bedside lockers had little in the way of possessions, so it was more a feeling that something was happening. While I felt by then that I had somewhat grasped their culture, the next 24 hours only reinforced my lack of understanding. It was the job of the midwives to manage the unit, but over time, we could only learn to respect a process that wasn't ours to control.

Our Aboriginal patients always had fond farewells. After all, we had nurtured them over a number of weeks. We saw many young teenage girls become women, as they had to start caring for their baby. I always hugged mother and baby and filled their small bag up with little extras they might need for bub.

Bessie was headed north towards her home – a 1000 kilometre journey that she had chosen to take without the RFDS. It wasn't uncommon for patients to make their own way home. There were always lifts along the way and extended family to see. Aboriginal women needed to reconnect with their land, and that wasn't possible in a cramped RFDS plane. They needed to feel the dirt between their toes again and smell the dry earth.

There was a quaint, old gold mining town 130 kilometres north of Kal that was home to many from the same desert tribal group as Bessie. Dawn is such a peaceful time of the day in the desert and this is when they found her. Just there on the outskirts of town, a dreadful violence had been committed against my patient. She had been murdered and the baby was found sucking at the breast.

That's what we were told. I was numb. I felt inadequate. Only the evening before, I had said goodbye and wished her well.

As health professionals we had a duty of care not to allow another operative delivery. This is because repeated Caesarean sections can weaken the uterus, increasing the risk of rupture. How difficult was it to bridge the cultural divide and obtain consent out there in the hot, dusty desert? The RFDS had done it many times over, but clearly, Bessie's husband wasn't in agreement. We were later told that her husband felt that his wife would be 'half a woman' after the sterilisation. In this patriarchal society the man regards his woman as his property. Did the loss of his wife's fertility prompt the ultimate act of domestic violence?

So, what was the role of the absconders? They knew that something grave was going to happen. Could any of them have prevented her murder? Was it because things within the family stay in the family? That it wasn't their role to intervene? That it was a deeply cultural issue that had imposed sanctions down to its very core? We never found out why they couldn't stop a murder. Over time, I've had to be courageous enough to accept the culture, their way of doing it. To learn that we don't always have the answers.

We were never told how the tribal elders ruled on this case, but the husband most probably would have been heavily dealt with by both cultures. That was the way it happened.

We had no formal debriefing of the kind they might do today. We were just left with our loss. Bessie's husband stayed in the desert during her confinement, as was common. We never met him. We were never told who raised the baby. We had to accept the unknowns.

Kalgoorlie came as a package for all us twenty-somethings living in the nurses' home. We had the time of our life, the price of gold doubled, and socially we never stopped to take a breath. And then something happened to burst that bubble and lay open issues we didn't know how to deal with. I felt a loss of innocence. I can't change what happened, but it has made me aware of the harsher elements of Aboriginal culture that midwives in the bush confront in the scope of their work. Twenty years on, and the stories from Kal still resonate in my head as well as my heart.

My coming and going from Kal was done on the train line. The staff from Maty stood out the back door as I farewelled Western Australia. I headed east, as our tears tumbled together on to the red earth.

Sage femme

HEATHER HARRIS

She's lying there, naked, sweat pouring down her face, and as each contraction engulfs her, she hits her hand against the tiled wall beside her – *slap, slap, slap slap SLAPSLAPSLAP slap slap slapslapslap . . . slap . . . slap . . . slap . . .*

The pain recedes and she rests, lying on her side, rocking slowly, eyes closed, black skin glistening.

It's June 2004, and I'm working as a midwife in the Ivory Coast in West Africa, at a small hospital near the Liberian border in a town called Danane. The Ivory Coast is at war with itself, torn along ethnic lines, and I'm here with Medecins Sans Frontières again, helping to care for the civilians caught up in this brutal affair. We are in rebel-held territory, so security is a little uncertain at times. There are guns and camouflage uniforms everywhere, the young soldiers dressed like gangsta rappers, but somehow I feel safe. Our hospital is the only one around and we deal with over 120 births a month, some very difficult, with no surgical facilities immediately available. The majority of babies are born in the villages and we never see them unless there is a problem.

The delivery room is small, with four delivery tables crammed into it. A woman lies on each one, in some stage of labour. At least they are separated by a plastic curtain – not that it's closed that often!

Jocelyne, a young Ivoirian *sage femme* (midwife, literally wise woman), is on duty today, but there are at least six other people in the room, some tending other labouring women, others whiling away their day off with their friends. There is little to do in this dusty little town when not needed for work. Midwives are highly respected here and are never called by their first name by those who are not their superior. It's always '*La sage*' which prefaces any request or remark. Usually, there is much chatter and general bonhomie.

But this woman is fully dilated, and has been for over two hours. She has been pushing for hours, but now she is exhausted and her baby's head is barely visible. The heat is tremendous and I'm sweating liberally. It drips on to the floor, and my glasses have drops running down inside them so that I can't see properly. I insert an IV and run some Ringers in to rehydrate her and perhaps encourage stronger contractions. We add some Syntocinon and wait for it to take effect.

Contractions start again, more insistent this time. The midwives and various other onlookers urge her on to greater efforts. The noise level rises further and voices become shrill.

'*Doucement! Doucement!*' I call, trying to quieten them a little and bring a little order into the apparent chaos. My French is not A1 and the fractured phrases I manage to put together are barely adequate, but everyone is patient with me and they try their best to understand.

The foetal heart rate is slowing; it clunks along at about 80. It's really time to get him out! There's no forceps here, the ventouse isn't working, exhortations to push are having little impact.

'*Pousse, pousse, pousse, ma cherie!*' Time to resort to a delivery method as old as childbirth itself. Pierrette, our youngest midwife, climbs on to the narrow bed and straddles the prostrate woman. Bintou, another cheerful and lovely *sage femme*, prods the uterus rhythmically, badgering it to start another contraction. As the uterus wearily tightens and bulges again, Pierrette forms her hands into fists and pushes, hard, hard, hard, on the pregnant fundus. The woman yells, moans, groans, pushes with her. I watch the head slowly advance, retreat, advance with each contraction.

Foetal heart is now 70. Stop listening, because there's nothing I can do except wait.

'Have the oxygen ready, get the ambubag, be ready with suction,' I instruct in my broken French. Another contraction, the head bulges on to the perineum . . .

'God, Jocelyne, what are you doing?!'

My newest *sage* stands waving a pair of scissors, about to cut into the thick, unstretched perineum.

'Wait, for God's sake!' I choke. 'Let's put some local in at least!'

Mercifully, episiotomies are very rarely made here and intact perineums are the norm. Although all the women are circumcised, it's not as radical as the procedure done in other African countries, and doesn't interfere with their birthing. I draw up the local anaesthetic and wait to numb the soft flesh. Another series of fundal pressures is applied. At long last, the blue head moves down, begins to crown. Jocelyne grabs a piece of the cloth the mother lies in and covers the bulging anus. Her sure little hands guide the expanding scalp over the taut perineum. The head seems to take forever to emerge! Long, moulded, covered in blood and meconium.

Now the bloody shoulders are stuck! Damn! Push the mother's legs back against her abdomen, scoop my finger in and hook the shoulder out . . . and finally his body slowly slides out. He is born.

'Scissors, *rapidement,* scissors! Where the hell are the bloody scissors!?'

The baby lies flaccid and pale on his mother's belly, making no effort to breathe at all.

'Clamp! Quick! Clamp! Scissors! Give me the cord ties. Where are the bloody scissors? Oh Christ – these blunt things? You could ride to London on these! *Commence l'oxygene! Ou est l'aspirateur?*'

The severed cord separates him from his mother and I lift his blue, limp body from her belly. I have him now, on the little trolley that serves so many purposes. The aspirator looks like a tiny turkey baster and isn't designed to clear anything except mouth and nose. We have to use what we've got, though, as there's nothing else.

Suck, suck.

'Give me the ambubag, the bloody ambubag – no, not that one, that's for adults. *Cherie, I need l'autre petite chose pour l'enfant!*'

God, why can't I speak French?

'*Merci. Commence reanimation, maintenant!*' It's all go go go, and our baby lies still, frail and unresponding.

'I need some adrenalin . . . no, no, no – *pas de problème*, there's a good heart rate. This bloody ambubag is useless! There's no air getting into his lungs.'

Although it's an emergency situation, somehow I don't feel panic. I suppose it's because I know there are few options in this stark environment, and the most basic resuscitation is all that is available. If the baby dies, the baby dies, but at least the mother is alive and well. It sounds so harsh, but that is how life is here.

'*Attend Maman.*'

It's Peggy, my most senior *sage femme*. She is a woman with a personality as big as her ample frame and I have the utmost respect for her capabilities. Although not yet 30, she has a depth of experience one can only get in an environment devoid of any of the technical wizardry we're used to in the West.

Her black hair is woven in tight corn-rows and she holds a Pinard's foetal stethoscope in her small, capable hand. She wraps some gauze over the flattened earpiece end. Then she places the open end over the baby's blue mouth and nose. She takes a deep breath and exhales forcefully down the Pinards. The baby's chest rises massively. All I can think is that he looks like a cane toad about to burst. God, I hope she doesn't blow his lungs up . . . Another big puff, and the stomach rises now.

I suddenly remember an old method of resuscitation I saw in a book from the early 1900s. I bend the baby's legs to his belly. Air gurgles out of his lungs, and his abdomen sinks. I straighten his legs and Peggy puffs again. I'm pushing blood back towards his heart, emptying his lungs and moving his diaphragm for him. We continue this archaic but effective resuscitation, while all around, voices buzz and other women continue labouring.

His colour is changing. He coughs and takes another breath, unaided. We massage up his back towards his heart and someone pours some cold Cetrimide on him. Again, a very routine way here to stimulate a newborn to cry. His arms fly out in shock and he cries in protest.

He has decided to stay. There is a general cheer of relief around the room and many '*Feliciations!*' The new mother is lying there beaming, relieved and thrilled that she has a live healthy baby to show for her tremendous effort.

This is about as basic as it gets. Birth and life, as rough and gritty as coarse gravel. Again I have learned something new to add to my repertoire. This is how it always is – with my years of Western experience, there is so much for me still to know.

I am privileged to be here. In the middle of a war zone, with no equipment and no technology, I see marvellous midwives applying their knowledge using their heads and their hands, plucking life from the jaws of death, making heroic efforts to save lives. We combine our collective wisdom, new and old, each learning from the other.

Suddenly my radio handset crackles and it is Radio Base asking if we have any emergency transfers. I look around the delivery room, at our newest baby, his relieved, exhausted mother, the other three women labouring, the two other pregnant women sitting in the corner waiting to be assessed.

I let the commotion roll off my shoulders and drip gently on to the floor.

'*Non, à e moment, c'est très normale!*' I reply, smiling.

Radio Base replies: '*Merci, terminé pour Radio Base.*'

Time for a cool drink and a five-minute break.

'*Merci,*' I reply. '*Terminé pour la salle d'accouchement.*'

BIRTH at HOME

Homebirth

ROBIN BARKER

Proserpine is hot and sunny. I spot Julia and Gabriel, hand in hand, just inside the terminal. Julia is smiling broadly. Behind the smile there's a shadow of late pregnancy weariness. Gabe looks healthy and energetic, full of beans. He's 23 months, sturdy and beautiful. White hair flops over his forehead and his face shows everything he's feeling. I could eat him.

We rattle out to LongGrass through the cane fields, very familiar to me now. Clunkety-clunk over the steel cattle grid before the steep drop into the creek bed.

We nose up the other side back on to the track and soon we're driving through the LongGrass gate into the clearing surrounded by rainforest where there's a fireplace, a rickety table, a couple of tree stumps and . . . a caravan. This time, instead of a tent, I have a caravan, courtesy of Michael's brother.

Cecil Rhodes, the Rhodesian ridgeback, lollops down to meet us. Cecil's put on weight and looks quite middle-aged. We greet each other woman to woman.

After unpacking I wander up to the house past the rainforest where tree roots hang suspended in great loops and the sunlight lands in intricate patterns on the forest floor. The house is built on a slope above the creek bed. One side is bound by the rainforest. On the other there's a cleared area of prickly grass with a vegie patch – tomatoes, basil, coriander – and a new white porcelain dunny sitting on a slab of concrete behind some bails of straw and a screen of bamboo. Swaying treetops surround the yard; beyond them, rows of blue hills fade into an even bluer sky.

That night, after Gabriel is asleep, we sit under mellow lights and eat vegetarian lasagne and drink a good red. Not Julia, I must hastily add – or at least, no more than a few mouthfuls.

'Eye contact, eye contact, eye contact,' we chant. We clink the glasses and ogle each other, eyes popping.

We don't know if the baby is a boy or a girl. General consensus among extended family members is leaning towards a boy. I'm undecided, and don't wish to commit myself.

'Indigo if it's a girl,' says Julia. 'That's certain. A boy . . . we're not so sure. Finn maybe, or Huon.'

We spend the evening reminiscing about Gabe's birth; the night skies as Mi and I drove home afterwards, the endless ruptured membranes and the bloody breastfeeding.

Gabe was born in hospital, mainly because Julia couldn't find a homebirth midwife, but halfway through this pregnancy she found Lou from Mackay. Lou has taken care of Julia since and is coming to LongGrass to help with the birth.

The next day we head off to Mackay to visit Lou in the new/old four-wheel drive, a Subaru covered in red dust, leaking a slow but persistent drop of water from somewhere underneath.

Mackay is a couple of hours' drive and it's peaceful bowling along in the sunshine talking about babies, births, relationships, writing and publishing gossip. What else is there of any importance?

We find Lou in the maternity section of the Mackay District Hospital, a crisp modern building with icy air-conditioning. She's dressed in shorts and sandals and looks cool and confident. She has strong bones and loose limbs, cropped hair and a big grin. She radiates capable calm, and I can see Julia unwind as Lou takes her blood pressure and talks about dates and possibilities. Julia lies on the bed and looks at the ceiling while Lou moves her hands over the bump, feeling the baby. She finds the heartbeat with the foetal monitor. We listen in silence to the thumpety-thump, a strong and healthy beat.

'The head's well down. We'll have a baby soon,' she says, pulling Julia up to sitting.

Julia and I feel reassured. We've been wondering what we'll do if my time at LongGrass comes and goes and Indigo/Huon still hasn't arrived.

By the time we get home Mi has fed Gabe, put him to bed and made the dinner. Later I make my way down to the caravan. Mi and Julia have left a small lantern near the bed, a candle enclosed in a glass cylinder. It is cosy and companionable with just enough light for me to read by. Outside, the night noises have started up. I wonder what's going on out there and feel I would like to join the party. All around me I hear scratching and scampering footsteps, sharp cries, snorting and digging sounds, and lots of thumping and heavy breathing, which I think might be the kangaroos getting it off.

Six days later I'm lying in bed dozing and listening to the birds, on the go since sunrise, when I hear Julia, Gabriel and Cecil coming down the track. Gabe clomps into the caravan in wellie-bobs and swarms all over the bed.

'Hey, Wobin . . . Hey, Wobin . . .' he keeps saying in a breathless voice but doesn't seem to know exactly what it is he wants to tell me.

Julia puts her head around the door. 'Membranes have ruptured. I'm leaking a bit.'

I peer around Gabe's squirming body. 'Much?'

She grimaces. 'No, just a trickle.'

'Any contractions?'

'Mild.'

We look at each other in silence.

'Coming for a walk?' Julia says.

'Sure, go ahead, wait at the gate. I'll catch you up.'

I duck outside for a pee. It's very early, the shadows are pale and long, the grass sharp and damp.

I join Julia and Gabe at the gate. We wander down the track past the liquid eyes and blunt faces of the neighbour's cows.

'I'll call Lou.'

'Definitely. Yes, call Lou.'

We both have a surge of comfort at the thought of Lou over there in Mackay. She'll know what to do.

After breakfast Julia calls Lou and her friend Alison, who has promised to mind Gabe during the birth. Lou is happy about the state of affairs – wait and see, and call her tomorrow – but Alison now has cystitis with a raging fever and isn't in any fit state to mind her own kids, let alone Gabe. A faint depression hovers. Gabe starts throwing scoops and diggers around the room.

'Just as well you're not in labour,' I say brightly. 'Twenty-four hours of antibiotics, and Alison will be okay.'

Julia nods slowly.

The day passes. I prepare tuna mornay for dinner. Cathy Freeman wins the 400 metres, which is fabulous for her but relatively unimportant to us. Julia folds and unfolds baby clothes.

The next morning Lou arrives early with an encouraging grin and a big blue suitcase. I peep into it when she opens it to get the foetal monitor and blood pressure machine. I'm amazed to see, among packets of dressings and instruments, a shower curtain. Julia is still losing some liquor, her blood pressure and temperature are fine, and Indigo/Huon's heartbeat is strong and hearty.

Everything starts to come together with Lou's arrival. She asks me to make sure dinner's ready ahead of time, so I'm at the stove as Lou and Julia sit at the table and discuss the castor oil in quiet voices.

Alison is over the worst of her cystitis, so Mi takes Gabe over to her place to spend the next 24 hours and arrives back with some cold stubbies in case anyone has the need of a beer. Sounds more agreeable to me than castor oil.

I have vague childhood memories of castor oil with sugar in it. The oil-soaked sugar granules used to get stuck on my tongue and in the crevices of my teeth. The taste stayed there for hours. I feel nauseated 50 years later just thinking about it.

'It has to be your decision,' Lou says. 'Eventually you'll come into labour, but the castor oil will almost certainly speed things along.'

Julia decides to go for the castor oil.

'It doesn't taste too good.' Lou is sympathetic. 'Mix it with orange juice and follow it up with a big drink of water.'

I have a photo of the castor oil moment. Through the window in the background sunlight is streaming down on to the deep green maze of the rainforest. In the foreground, Julia cracks a smile with the look of a child about to jump off a diving board for the first time. Lou peers out with an impish grin as she mixes up the castor oil and orange juice in a tall glass.

Julia drinks the castor oil in one gulp, then we all stand and look at her, waiting for something to happen. Suddenly we don't have anything to do.

Gabe's away, dinner's ready, the beer is cold, but . . . the washing's still on the line. While I'm out the back yanking nappies down, God speaks to me. She tells me the baby is a girl. When I go back inside, Lou is tidying up and organising her things for a swim.

I dump the clothes on the bed and fold up the washing. 'It's a girl. A voice spoke to me out at the clothesline. It was very clear – it's a girl, Indigo.'

Mi, Julia and Lou look at me doubtfully. Really?

Lou pops the castor oil in the big blue suitcase lying on the seat under the window, sweeps her eyes over the contents one last time, then clicks it shut. 'Rob and I will leave you two for a while. We'll go for a swim and pick up a few things in Proserpine. By the time we get back, things will be on the move.'

When we pull up near the caravan after our swim and a trip to the bottle shop at Proserpine for a few bottles of red, we hear the deep growl of a cello.

'Sounds promising,' Lou says as we walk up to the house.

Inside, Julia is on her journey. She walks back and forth, her face absorbed and serious.

'That's taken the smile off her face,' Lou whispers.

We sit and watch Julia, naked, walking with fearsome concentration, focused on something we can't see or hear. The vibrations of the cello music bounce off the timber floor. Outside I can hear the wind in the trees, the thrum of the crickets, and the sounds of Cecil flopping and scratching around the deck.

There's nothing fluttery or vague about these contractions now. They have a distinct rhythm and come every few minutes with their own narrative shape. Julia has to stay on her feet and keep mobile – it's too painful for her to do anything else. Lou shows Michael how to bend forward so that Julia can rest on his back during contractions.

'And Rob,' she says. 'I want you to be responsible for a warm flannel for the perineum. It needs to be good and warm, but not hot. I'll tell you when.'

I immediately put the kettle on so I won't be caught short, then sit at the table with Mi. He has a pencil behind his ear. From time to time he scribbles in an exercise book while he sips on a coldie. Lou sits on the window seat near the blue suitcase. She is so tuned into Julia's body she seems to know exactly what is going on without talking or moving from her position by the window. There is little conversation. We concentrate on each other, exchanging glances like a string quartet waiting for the next cue.

Two hours slip away. Julia keeps walking. Her control is astonishing. The next contraction is more intense. Lou presses a cold flannel to Julia's forehead, anchors her with her eyes for 30 seconds, then goes back to her seat by the window.

Julia has been walking now for four-and-a-half hours. She has a faint smile. 'What's happened to the music?'

I leap to my feet. 'I'll put something on. What do you want?'

'How about the Wiggles?' Mi says, taking a mouthful of beer, and we laugh.

Julia isn't amused. 'That's not funny, Michael . . .' She sways and moans softly.

Lou squats under Julia's legs, looks up and nods. She snaps open the locks of the suitcase, spreads the shower curtain on the bed and lays out some instruments.

I feel light-headed, a little dizzy. I've been waiting for the opening of the suitcase for the last hour. I think from the look of relief on Michael's face that he's been waiting as well. A stream of liquid splatters on to the floor with the next contraction. Somehow Lou manages to mop up and help Julia on to the bed all at the same time. Julia kneels on the bed with her bum in the air. I reheat the water and join Mi and Lou at the foot of the bed. Lou pulls on a pair of gloves and talks quietly to Julia who gives gentle persuasive pushes with each contraction. I know it must be hurting like hell, that burning sensation as the perineum stretches, but the only sounds she makes are little rhythmic gasps as the baby's head starts to appear.

'Hot cloth, Rob,' Lou calls.

Oh, my God, I've forgotten about the hot cloth, the only thing I have to do. I dash to the kettle and pour boiling water on to the flannel. It's way too hot. Julia would have a scarred fanny for life if Lou wacked that on to her perineum.

I put it under the cold-water tap but the water flow at LongGrass isn't much more than a steady drip. I let the water trickle over the flannel, shake it and wave it and stick it under the water again. Luckily, Lou seems to be involved in something else momentarily.

'Got that cloth, Rob?'

'Coming.' I walk across the room flapping it to and fro.

It's a nice warm heat by the time Lou presses it against Julia's perineum.

I remember the camera and grab it as the baby's head is born, slowly, contraction by contraction.

'Round here, Michael,' says Lou. 'You do the catching.'

Mi stands waiting with one hand cupped under the curve of the baby's head. A perfect face – with puffy eyes jammed shut, a button nose and plump purple lips – pokes out from between Julia's buttocks. Julia breathes heavily and makes small grunting sounds. The baby starts to cry. It's a tentative wail to begin with, then gets louder, more confident. Mi's eyes are wet, his face shifting from ecstasy to concern. Lou waits for the baby's shoulders to rotate with the next contraction. It seems to take an eternity. When the contraction comes, the shoulders slip out and Indigo glides down into her father's waiting hands.

'It's a girl, Julia, a girl. I knew it was.' I do some childlike leaps and take her hand.

She is pale with exhaustion, but her eyes are bright. She smiles and squeezes my fingers. 'I'm really glad you were here.'

Mi passes Indigo through Julia's legs, the glistening blue cord trailing behind like an abseiler's rope. With one graceful move, Julia sits back on her haunches and lifts Indigo off the bed. They gaze into each other's eyes.

Indigo's skin is multi-hued; navy, dark red and pink, with patches of bright red. Her feet and hands are deeply creased, lavender-tinged. Soon Julia is propped up against the wall with Indigo cradled in her arms while Mi cuts the cord under instruction from Lou.

We all feel euphoric. The room is full of laughter and warmth. Sometime later Julia has another small contraction, there's a rush of blood and the placenta slips out with a squelch. It's half-past four.

Over the next hour Lou weighs and measures Indigo, dresses her in warm clothes, wraps her in three cuddlies and puts an oversize beanie on her head. She looks like a comical pastry chef peeping over the top of the cuddlies with one eye open and one eye shut.

Lou helps Julia down to the shower. Outside the sunlight is fading, and it's mild and still. Small birds gather and whirl about, spreading the news. I watch Lou take care of Julia at the shower, soaping her up, rinsing her off. I look around the house.

Apart from the bundle Mi holds in his arms, it's hard to know a birth has just taken place.

My memories of hospital births are of piles of bloody linen, bundles of instruments and tubing, bottles of white antiseptic cream on stainless steel trolleys, and overflowing bins.

Here, I hold Indigo for a few minutes. She is as firm as a peach. She grunts, her face goes red, and a big earthy shit oozes out from the sides of her nappy. It sticks to her legs like tar.

It's eight o'clock and we're sitting around the table shovelling down lentils, drinking red wine, swapping notes, all as high as kites. Michael's nose is red, his eyes look crossed. Julia is at a point somewhere between comatose and delirium. I feel very weak and keep collapsing into paroxysms of uncontrollable giggles.

Lou looks as fresh as a daisy. 'I could tell the minute we walked back in that you were in labour, Julia – no smile,' she says.

'I was worried you mightn't get back in time,' Julia replies. 'In fact, I think I was starting to get a little cross.'

Lou chortles. 'Haven't missed one yet.'

'I was so relieved, Lou, when you went to the blue suitcase and opened it up . . .' I say, remembering.

'Yes . . .' Michael and Julia chorus. 'The blue suitcase!'

A gust of laughter breaks out all round.

'You're amazing, Stiles,' Mi says softly to Julia.

Someone proposes a toast. 'Eye contact, eye contact, eye contact,' we chorus.

We raise our glasses, push our faces forward and eyeball each other wildly. Julia looks as if she's about to fall off the chair. Lou bundles mother and baby off to bed, while Michael and I clear up the dishes. One by one we give Julia and Indigo a kiss before we head off to the clearing below the house where Michael has the fire going. We sit in the moonlight, slightly stunned. A light breeze sends bursts of sparks up from the fire into a sky full of stars.

Michael lights a cigar and takes a swig of malt whisky. Lou opens a packet of fags and looks at me cautiously.

'Only occasionally,' she says. 'You know – to celebrate.'

I laugh. 'Lou, I'd love a celebratory fag if you've got one to spare.'

She chucks me the packet.

'Are all homebirths like that?' I ask, inhaling. The rush of nicotine makes my head spin pleasantly.

Lou nods. 'More or less.'

'Julia was so brave,' I say. 'So controlled.'

The homebirth alternative wasn't available in my day, but I doubt I'd have had the capacity to pull it off. At the time, I remember, I was rather keen on the idea of chemical pain relief.

We shift into a drowsy, murmuring conversation that drifts in unfinished sentences across the fire.

Lou stands and stretches. 'I'm off to bed. I have to get back to Mackay first thing.'

A few days later, my time is up. I'm having cosy time with Indigo before Mi takes me to the airport. I cradle her head in my hand and breathe in her warm baby scent. Her cheek is against mine, smooth as satin.

Suddenly it's time. One last photo. Mi fixes the camera up on the kitchen bench, then runs back to join us. I hold Gabe. We all beam. A quick flash, kisses, hugs and watery eyes before Mi and I head down the track.

I look back as I close the gate. Beautiful LongGrass. It's not an easy life here. I don't think Mi and Julia will realise just how tough it is until years down the track, but I know the memories will be sweet.

Sweet, hilarious, sun-blessed.

Breakfast at Simone's

BRONNI HAWKSWORTH

'Hello, Bronni. It's Simone. The baby, it's coming today. Do you think it would be a good day for you?'

So typical of Simone to ask. She's worried that I need to organise my children, while she's having those gentle first contractions of labour.

Me? I'm ecstatic. My wedding anniversary is tomorrow and now I know I won't be on call for it.

I jump in the shower and try to arrange my 'midwife head', as the adrenalin and sheer joy that it's all worked out perfectly, again, courses through my veins.

'Damn, I must get myself that non-spill cup,' I think as I struggle out the door in the dark, trying not to wake the kids.

The moon is in almost full splendour to the west as I drive through the hills. It's February, but it's unusually cold. So, the weatherman had actually been right, correctly predicting the need for extra blankets tonight. *100, 100, just stick to the speed limit, my girl. You'll be there in plenty of time.*

The house is bathed in candlelight, inviting in the good spirits, and the fire is ablaze. These are some of the nicest things about having babies at home. Eberhard seems more comfortable now that I'm here. *This is woman's business*, he says with all his actions. An old-school German man with the integrity of a big, strong, calm ox. He puts on rice for breakfast and checks on the kids. Simone is excited, but still unsure. Even with child number four, early labour is still a time of great adjustment.

Jennie arrives and we are complete. Let's just hope that Jennie's other woman doesn't get into cracking labour just yet! It's all about trust. Always.

Jennie's mobile rings and she slips out to the verandah to take the call. Simone looks into my eyes. 'My waters have broken – but, well, they still are only little.' My excitement is beaming through my eyes at her, I know. 'Shall we let the chooks out?' she says.

Being outside is good for Simone. She gathers herself as she says goodnight to the moon and greets the day.

'Let's walk.'

She can't stop talking and giggles with embarrassment at the life story that comes tumbling out. East Germany was so different, with pain a part of her daily life. Now here she is pain-free (contractions excepted) and living in a land of plenty. My respect for her and her family grows with each story I hear.

We're at the end of the road and now it's uphill all the way back. The contractions are gently increasing in intensity but we are just enjoying the space. A mother of three beautiful children already, Simone knows this time is precious – this stillness before the journey of chaos and love that a new babe brings.

The white rabbit comes out of nowhere, like we were in a Lewis Carroll book. We stop and watch, then greet a neighbour as politely as we could considering Simone's embarrassment at being caught outside in Eberhard's flannel work shirt. Another contraction and it's time to head home. You know when it's just not right to be away anymore.

Johannes, the youngest, is up, but Eberhard manages to settle him down again. You can see Simone relax a little with her babe happily back in slumberland. She's exhausted after being awake all night, but the contractions are getting stronger. Eberhard's got breakfast organised. The rice, fruit, nuts and soymilk are warm and comforting. Jennie and I realise we had better eat now. Things are moving along.

Simone's birth song wakes the girls and, wide-eyed, they creep downstairs. Today is the day that Mum's been saying will come. Eberhard organises their clothes and brekky. Jennie and I take turns to be with Simone at each contraction and finish breakfast at the same time. I love the way Jennie and I work together. We have a rhythmic dance that we surround Simone with without saying a word.

Even when Johannes wakes, things remain calm and reverent. Children know in their bones just what is going on, and at two years Johannes isn't the least bit perturbed and is demanding his breakfast now.

The girls are starting to sense a change in the intensity and move to sit on the lounge room floor behind Mum while Jennie and I stand either side. Simone is standing, leaning and squatting and singing her beautiful song. Even the gentlest women get to that place of pure strength as full opening approaches. She slips into pushing in a contraction, and Jennie pops down on her knees while I stay to soothe Simone with a cold face washer and whisper love and encouragement. Gently Jennie speaks to Simone. 'Just breathe this bit out. You're doing so well.'

The children (Johannes has had enough of breakfast now) are awe-struck by the amazing face that is sitting between Mum's legs. Simone reaches down with the next contraction and takes her baby into her arms and sits to a squat. There are cries of joy and love and tears and kisses and much excitement.

'Oh, it's a boy!' Eberhard moves over to see his son. He is proud and his words of love for his wife will be spoken when they are alone as a family.

Jennie and I retreat, holding the space at a distance. We kiss and hug and glow with the joy of life. We are ourselves, yet again, blown away by the journey of women.

Simone needs to move and, with her entourage of glowing faces, we hold her elbows as she strides to the fire. She rests here for a while, reliving her journey. Only now can she speak of her time. Her babe is awake and staring intently at his mother, listening with all the wisdom of the world to his birth story.

Wrapped in her dressing gown, babe in her arms, her man at her side, and nappy over the loo, Simone delivers her placenta. Oh, it is so beautiful. The children are keen to see where their brother was hiding in Mum's womb.

'Wow! The bag that held the waters is so thin, and there's two thin bits, and look it's like a tree – a blue and red tree.'

It's time for school, and Johannes decides he wants to go with Dad. There is much instruction in German, and bag grabbing and kissing to go around and once again peace descends. A woman, her babe, her midwives. There is nothing more ancient.

With only the slightest instruction from us, Simone washes her babe's placenta with exquisite tenderness. She chats gaily about how she didn't expect it to feel so beautiful, so normal. For Jennie and me, no interruption of the all-important third stage, and no cutting of the cord (lotus birth), is a joy we get to experience so often. Tucking the lovingly wrapped placenta in with her babe, Simone gathers the two and they snuggle in for a feed.

She knows she should eat, but can't. She knows she should sleep, but won't. She just gazes, offers more breast and gazes again. Johannes is back and is so big all of a sudden. Relegated to toddlerhood overnight, so grown up, so loud. His egocentric way is a wonderful reality check for the weeks to come.

The bloodstained sheets are in the basin soaking. A load is on in the washing machine. Jennie and I gather our equipment, which all of a sudden looks so clinical and unnecessary, but which has brought us great strength in the past. Another cuppa and scheduling for visits. Simone is tucked up and Eberhard is bustling about. Already friends have started the food tree that means much support for the family in this strong, supportive community. More hugs and tears, and before we know it we're off again into the big wide world.

Did the world look this beautiful yesterday? Knowing I will be holding the space for mother and babe for the next few days, I call in to see my women friends. We sit around in a circle. We cry tears of joy to hear of another woman's power story and we celebrate a woman and babe as we celebrate all women and their babes. The sharing of stories and food, and I am once again refilled.

It's not easy being a mother and midwife, but there is nothing else worth doing.

A bush birth

MONICA FEDER

I didn't want to go to work. The centre had been so quiet during December, I imagined that no onc would want to see a maternal and child health nurse the first day back from the Christmas/New Year break. In such a small country town, why would they need me?

'You'll be right when you get there,' said my husband when he saw my long face, trying to cheer me up. To make myself feel a bit better, I threw on my lovely Laura Ashley scarf a girlfriend had given me for Christmas.

I drive the 80 kilometres to the little rural town, but I still don't want to go to the cold, lonely centre. I drop in on the girls in the community health centre on the edge of town for a chat and some company. The nurses are busy seeing patients behind closed doors, so the receptionist and I chat about our respective Christmases and the 'joys' of being back at work. Finally I can delay no longer, and I get back into the car to drive down to the little maternal and child health centre, nestled between the public hall and the public toilets.

I unlock the door, open the blinds and turn on the heating. 'Ridiculous,' I think. 'It's January in the Wimmera and I'm turning on the heaters.'

As I reach to check the message bank the phone rings. It's the same receptionist I was laughing with only minutes earlier.

'What's wrong, Joy?' I say. 'I was only just talking to you.'

'There's a lady having a baby at home NOW and we need your help.'

I gasp as my heart leaps to my throat, and my Laura Ashley scarf slips from my shoulders. 'Where is she?' I splutter.

Joy begins to give me detailed directions to a farmhouse out of town, then stops mid-sentence. 'Don't worry,' she says. 'Pam's on her way and will pick you up.'

Now what do I do? To say that I'm panic-stricken is an understatement! I run from the phone to the storage cupboards under the sink; God only knows why. What would I find in there to assist with a birth, among the old dusty Christmas decorations, coffee jars and spare immunisation supplies? I race back to the phone and pick it up. Why? Who will I call: 'Dial a Birth'? What's the point? In the following fifteen seconds I grab the first aid kit from the car boot and the Air-Viva bag and mask, then run down to the service station to tell the owner there is an emergency. I ask her to put a note on the door instructing any mothers who arrive to leave their names and I'll ring them later.

Where is Pam, where is she? I need her now! I don't know what sort of car she'll be driving. Come to think of it, I don't even know Pam! I guess she'll be the one who comes roaring up the road at breakneck speed, as desperate to see me as I am to see her.

Pam soon pulls up and I try to jump in, but she's got the 'Emergency Folder for Rural Nurses' taking up the whole front seat. I grab it and throw it in the back. 'We haven't got time for any reading, Pam. Just drive!'

Pam isn't a midwife, and is very anxious. 'Thank God it's Wednesday and you're in town,' she keeps saying.

'Thank God you're working today and know where this family lives,' I reply.

As we negotiate the dirt track to the farmhouse I try to refresh every principle and complication I've ever learned about childbirth. It's only been ten months since I worked in mid, but 'Compromised Childbearing' at uni never really covered bush births in remote rural locations.

We pull into the driveway. There is the sound of a small dog yap, yap, yapping. There are two cars already there with doors flung open, and the garden gate hangs open in welcome. I grab the first-aid kit and leap from the car before Pam has come to a full stop.

At the gate I see that I won't even need to go inside. Kerry, Grant and a new baby are on the back open verandah awaiting our arrival! Mum is on all fours with her clothing askew, while Dad is holding a wet, blue, shivering baby between Mum's legs. I'm not sure if the baby is shivering himself, or merely shaking because his father's hands are! Kerry, the mother, is vague, dazed and cold. She is shivering but says that her legs are stiff from maintaining her 'all fours' position – she has been too frightened to move.

With very brief introductions I throw open the first-aid kit, hoping that a cord clamp and sterile scissors will be sitting on top. No such luck, of course. There's a small towel which I spread on the verandah as I rummage through the kit looking for something to 'disconnect' mother and child. Right, ribbon gauze! That will be the cord clamp. Clean scissors! They will do just nicely. I wind the ribbon around the cord a few times and tie it tight, then repeat the process. I delegate Pam to look after the mother while I look after bub. I think about asking Dad to cut the cord, but I think he's done enough! He seems very relieved that the 'troops' have arrived.

I cut the cord, sweep the baby up, clutch him to my chest and stride through the kitchen door.

There is an older woman standing there who introduces herself as Janet, the children's nanna. She'd planned to look after the two older children while her son took his wife to hospital, but things had gone a little too fast. I ask her for plenty of towels. The baby is large – about 8 pounds I imagine – and he is breathing, cold to the touch and quite blue.

The towels arrive and I immediately start giving the little man a vigorous rub. He doesn't like it and gives a lusty yell, filling his lungs with oxygen and turning his torso a lovely healthy shade of pink. His dad comes in when he hears the noise.

'He's alright, isn't he?' he asks.

'He's fine,' I reply.

He gives me a quick impulsive bear hug as I juggle his baby, a hug of relief and gratitude. The tears start to fill my eyes. But they're not flowing yet – there's more work to do. I call Nanna again, this time to ask for singlets, jumpsuit, beanie and bunny rugs. She has the carefully packed suitcase on the floor and quickly finds what we need.

I ask the two small girls in the lounge room if they want to see their new brother, but the TV is on and *Play School* is just too important.

I dress the baby, wrapping him well in the bunny rugs, and give him to his nanna to cuddle and keep warm while I go back out to check on Mum.

Pam and I bring her inside and help her get comfortable in bed. I'm just palpating her fundus, preparing her for the third stage of labour when the 'ambos' arrive. I peek out of the bedroom and am greeted by two volunteer ambulance officers, Ken and Cameron, in their overalls. They're both wearing smiles as broad as a Wimmera sunset.

'Well, well. What have we here?' Ken asks. 'A homebirth! What do you want us to do?'

I giggle to myself. I can see they're both enjoying this experience, so removed from their normal call of duty.

'Well, you could boil the water. That hasn't been done yet,' I reply. Without a word they turn on their heels and head to the kitchen. I know I probably shouldn't be so cheeky, but there's no need for them to observe the third stage, is there?

With the placenta delivered and secure in a plastic bag, I help Kerry with a shower. This finally gives us time for a chat about the circumstances leading up to the baby's birth. She tells me she slept poorly the night before and had been up to the toilet a few times with diarrhoea. The last visit to the toilet had led to four contractions. She had a doctor's appointment scheduled for later that morning and thought the timing was ideal, not thinking that she could already be in labour. She'd rung Grant to tell him about the contractions and ask him to accompany her to the doctor's. Not long after he'd arrived home, her membranes had ruptured and suddenly the baby's head was on view!

I come out of the bathroom to find Grant, as Kerry needs some fresh clothes. He hands me a dress which I pass on to Kerry in the bathroom. I'm greeted in the hallway with a great ruckus as the ambos try to manoeuvre the trolley into the house.

'No need for that,' I say. 'This woman is quite capable of walking the few yards to the ambulance.' The ambos look puzzled at this. Patients don't usually walk to their own ambulances, do they?

Kerry is trying to button the dress but has no hope; it's one of her pre-pregnancy outfits and there is no way it will button across the chest. We find something a bit more suitable and take a few quick photos of the family on the couch before it's time to load one and all into the ambulance. First, Kerry is made comfortable with plenty of blankets against the cold wind. I'm impatient for them to get moving, as I can see a band of dark, sinister clouds to the west, and the dirt road looks like it would soon get slippery with a shower of rain. Once the suitcase is in the car, and the placenta stored in the ambulance, I run to fetch the still unnamed infant. The rain is starting.

I hold the little boy to my chest, throw a single bed blanket over both our heads and make a run for it as those big cold drops fall.

When both mother and child are loaded, Ken closes the door.

'By the way,' he says, turning to me. 'That water has boiled. What do you want me to do with it?'

I'm back at the door of the house by now. 'MAKE THE TEA, OF COURSE!' I yell back to him with a big grin. 'Don't you think we deserve it?'

'You're right, love!' He grins back at me. 'Have one for me, too!'

I ring the midwifery ward to hand over, then Pam, Janet and I sit down to that cup of tea at the table that, less than an hour before, had been a makeshift resuscitation cot. Together, we have a good laugh and a debrief. Janet tells us that she had called the ambulance and community health centre, as Grant was helping Kerry. She, too, had been shocked at the pace at which everything had happened. The baby has yet to be named, but she promises to ring us later and tell us what Kerry and Grant choose. She is so grateful for our assistance and thanks us many times, but I keep thanking her in return – for keeping a cool head, getting what was requested without question, and holding the baby to keep him warm.

Just another day at the office. How am I going to focus and finish the day back at the centre after a buzz like that?

I saw Kerry a week later for her and baby Karl's first official maternal and child health home visit. Kerry's return home was delayed, as Karl had developed jaundice and had required five days of phototherapy. The doctors had told her that this was due to his rapid birth and that his face was quite bruised. Kerry also spoke of the bumpy, fast ride in the ambulance. At one stage she had called out to Ken to slow down, as she feared that she was going to be bounced off the ambulance stretcher.

At the hospital Kerry had felt quite the celebrity, as there was a welcoming committee of about six Accident and Emergency staff all standing there grinning and saying 'Congratulations', directing her straight through to mid.

When her GP, a man not normally noted for his sense of humour, came in to see her, he'd told her that if she was thinking of having another baby she was to pitch a tent on the hospital grounds two weeks before her due date.

I know that the chances of there being another birth like this are quite remote, but I'm not going to get caught again. Now in my car's first-aid kit, at the very top, are two sterile cord clamps. No need for ribbon gauze next time. Pity I haven't got room for the kettle . . .

Stuck shoulders

JAN ROBINSON

When a partly born baby cannot continue its journey because of stuck shoulders, I always encourage the labouring woman to respond to the signals her baby is sending. This way, the woman deals with the situation herself, adjusting the posture of her trunk and pelvis to dislodge the offending shoulders. However, this particular episode was the most frightening of my career – as the mother, Shirley, collapsed with exhaustion after valiantly struggling to push out her baby's shoulders. This left me working through every rescue manoeuvre I knew, for what seemed like forever, until eventually the poor little mite was released from his tight-fitting trap.

Shirley and her husband, Duncan, had been up until well after midnight attending to the final editing and collation of a book Shirley was writing. They finally sank into bed exhausted after meeting the publisher's deadline. As is often the case when parents get to bed very late, the children wake up early! Ten-year-old Callum and seven-year-old Lachlan were just winding up for the day with a musical rendition for their mother (they were both learning different instruments) when it occurred to Shirley that her labour might be starting. The boys were very excited, as each had a special list of 'jobs' planned to help their mother and father during the labour and birth.

When Shirley called me later that day I lost no time in getting to her home. More often than not, large babies seem to arrive quickly and this baby had felt quite a good size when I last palpated.

Shirley's contractions were becoming strong and regular when I arrived that afternoon. She looked absolutely exhausted, but said she was okay. 'I'm past the point of being able to lie down and rest anyway,' she said. Once Shirley heard her baby's heartbeat, she smiled. I reassured her that the baby sounded very happy despite the strengthening contractions. Slowly she ate a small piece of apple and then focused on her baby and surrendered to her labour.

Duncan and the boys had finished filling the pool, so early that evening Shirley moved into the water to give birth. She was kneeling and leaning forward with her head resting on the side of the pool. She worked nicely with her contractions, letting her body relax and letting her baby move down a little with each one. Eventually I saw part of the baby's head appear beneath the water. After a few more contractions the head slowly crowned and I checked the foetal heartbeat for the last time – steady at a normal rate.

'The head should be free with the next contraction,' I said to Shirley, smiling.

But it wasn't. It took two more contractions for the head to be slowly born almost to the chin, which didn't free itself. This 'turtle-neck' sign rang the warning bells in my head. Could this baby's shoulders be stuck high in the birth canal?

'Don't panic. Shirley's trunk is upright! She's bringing her knee up spontaneously. She can do this!' I repeated to myself. But three more strong contractions with all of Shirley's energy going into them followed, and there was still no movement of the baby's head. No turning, no progress forward, despite her herculean efforts.

Shirley, a petite woman, was by now looking extremely vulnerable and exhausted squatting in the middle of the pool. She moved over to the edge, leaned forward and rested her head on Duncan's strong thighs. Callum and Lachlan, not suspecting anything was wrong, had their camera and tape recorder ready to roll.

I decided I had best get into the water. The colour of the baby's head looked fine underwater, so I realised there was no undue pressure on the baby's cord. I didn't attempt to feel around the baby's neck, as this action would have caused Shirley terrible pain. I asked her permission to try and 'jiggle' the baby's head (similar to easing a tight cork out of a bottle) with the next contraction. I explained that performing this action might startle the baby into trying to breathe, so it would mean an end to the underwater birth plans.

Shirley struggled to stand up and lean over Duncan's strong shoulders. She brought her right knee up as high as she could, resting her foot on the side of the pool.

With the next contraction she pulled down on Duncan's neck, bringing her buttocks down while I gently moved the baby's head from side to side. Shirley was using all her might, but still nothing happened! By now the warning bells were louder, accompanied by flashing lights inside my head. Everyone in the room knew it – this baby was well and truly stuck!

Shoulder dystocia.

I needed to start further manoeuvres, and quickly. Shirley sensed the urgency of the situation and hung off Duncan's neck again. Duncan was her rock, moving in synchronisation with her every effort. She was able to maintain a supported squat while pushing with her next contraction . . . and still nothing happened.

I asked Shirley to bring her knees up higher with the next contraction, and after it she was red in the face from pushing. As the contraction ended she flopped down on to the floor, almost on top of the baby's head.

'I can't help you any more, Jan,' she gasped, so exhausted she was almost semi-conscious. I asked Callum and Lachlan to keep their eyes on the clock, thinking we should be able to free the baby after the next contraction. Duncan and I positioned Shirley on the floor with her head angled forward and Duncan holding her knees back on to her chest. Shirley's thighs were abducted with the next contraction while I exerted the strongest pressure that I could over the baby's shoulder, positioned just above her pubic bone. Shirley continued to push with all her might, while I strained to push down the shoulder. Nothing.

By this time eight minutes had passed, so I asked Callum to call an ambulance. Even if I got the baby out before it arrived, we might still need help with resuscitation.

The baby's head still remained a reasonable colour, but I was worried that this might change and lead to oxygen deprivation. I had terrible visions of transporting Shirley to the nearest hospital with an incompletely born baby. I could vaguely hear Callum talking to the ambulance people. He sounded so calm, giving concise and accurate directions over the telephone.

My mind was racing! Mentally, I began revising all the shoulder dystocia manoeuvres I'd ever learned. I still hadn't tried turning Shirley on her side with her knees tucked up into her chest. This so-called foetal position, which most of us use to drift off to sleep, isn't so comfortable when one still has most of a large baby and placenta still inside one's abdomen.

Shirley, now in a mild state of shock, was incapable of helping. Duncan once again changed her position, and I can remember being so thankful for his size and strength and his gentleness with Shirley. While he kept Shirley's knees up, I continued to gently move the baby's head from side to side. There was still no movement and I knew there was no more that I could do other than to perform an invasive procedure by entering the birth canal and trying to 'corkscrew' the baby around, to encourage the stuck shoulder to rotate to the front where it might slide down behind the pubic bone and, finally, into the pelvis.

I quickly washed my gloved hand (no time to open antiseptics now), explaining to Duncan what I would have to do. He did his part by keeping Shirley's knees up and ensuring she was breathing. Amazingly, the baby's head still looked a reasonable colour. But I didn't have time to listen to foetal heart sounds again. By now

I could feel my own heart racing, although the bells and lights had stopped filling my head.

I began by placing my fingers along the back of the baby's neck and slid them upwards. I felt Shirley's perineum tear. Lachlan was pouring the antiseptic cream over my hand (under his father's directions, bless him) as I moved my searching fingers ever so slowly. At last I located the offending posterior shoulder and realised that the arm attached to it was high up at the level of Shirley's abdomen. But I could splint the arm with my fingers! Using it as a lever I began to sweep the arm across the baby's chest. At the same time the baby's body began to turn to the front.

I felt something 'give' inside. Fear that I had fractured the baby's collarbone filled me. But rotating the baby had freed the shoulder, albeit now dislocated, allowing a very limp, discoloured baby boy to slip into the world straight into a pool of his mother's blood. Shirley's perineum had torn deeply – the episiotomy scar she'd incurred with Callum's birth had opened up and was now bleeding profusely. I quickly grabbed a sterile sponge and compressed it into the wound to stem the bleeding, and congratulated Shirley on her new baby boy.

I'm not sure that she heard me. I was now busy puffing oxygen into the baby, and I gave him an Apgar score of two; one for some colour and one for a heart beat. He was deeply shocked, but unbelievably, his cord was still pulsating!

Despite everything, the placenta hadn't separated. Wonderful! At least he was getting some oxygen from the placenta as I continued puffing oxygen into his lungs to remind him to breathe. I heaved a sigh of relief as I heard the boys letting the ambulance officers through the front door. Callum told me it was fifteen minutes since the baby's head had come out. He had written down all the times, as asked. Usually a baby is completely born during the next one or two contractions after the birth of the head. Fifteen minutes was the longest birth interval I have ever been associated with.

Shirley was slowly coming around and apologising for causing so much trouble. The first ambulance officer could see that I knew what I was doing, and offered to take Shirley's vital signs as I continued to resuscitate the baby. I wished that I had Shirley's strength as she began to regain her colour and pick up her energy. I wondered why mothers always blame themselves when things don't go to plan. I reassured Shirley that this unexpected challenge was none of her doing. At the same time, I was looking at Duncan's giant frame and deciding that this rather large baby had more than likely inherited his father's genetic make-up!

The strong little baby boy slowly responded and regained some muscle tone. We all heard a small 'sigh' come from him. Within a few minutes his colour began to improve. When he was finally breathing without assistance I left the oxygen blowing over his face for a few more minutes while I dried him thoroughly, wrapping him in the warm wrap fetched by Lachlan.

Duncan held and kept his newborn son warm while Shirley drank a few sips of warm water, brought to her by Callum. She then made one last supported squat and delivered her placenta. The second ambulance officer had assured us he could 'do an active third stage' and was dying to do it all for her, but Shirley showed us all what amazing strength unmedicated birthing women possess.

Both ambulance officers acknowledged they had never seen anyone deliver their own placenta before and were in awe of Shirley doing this just after recovering from such a shocking experience.

We made Shirley comfortable while we discussed the options for the baby's ongoing care. As it was now past midnight, I knew there would be no newborn baby specialist on duty at the local hospital and we didn't relish the thought of a baby recovering from shock spending the rest of the night waiting among a lot of sick people as one was called in. We declined the ambulance officers' offer to take us, as the paediatric consultation was no longer urgent – the baby's colour and breathing were now okay. We could all sense his pain, though, when his damaged arm was touched or moved. I made a sling for the limp arm and pinned it to the baby's other shoulder for comfort and to avoid further damage.

Duncan and Shirley announced that the baby was to be named Alistair, and his brothers each had a short time holding him and comforting him carefully while their father made a meal. As he did so, I began to repair Shirley's perineum. She made the tedious task of stitching easier for me, using this time we had together to ask lots of questions about the long delay with Alistair's birth. I felt terrible that I had torn the old episiotomy scar, but Shirley told me that it had opened up with Lachlan's birth.

Alistair was showing some interest in feeding after a few hours' rest, and despite his damaged arm we managed not to hurt him too much when putting him to the breast. After some debriefing with the boys, Duncan put them to bed. Finally, Shirley and Alistair were ready to settle down for a well-earned rest. I tucked mother and baby in together and let myself out of the house, promising to be back after I had a few hours' sleep myself.

Normally as I drive home from a birth I do a 'victory cry and gesture' when I pass another vehicle. This time, as I passed the only truck on the road, I was so speechless and drained I could do neither. I realised how close it had been for Alistair.

After I arrived home, I knew that I had to debrief with someone other than my dog. It was just dawn, but I had to talk to another midwife. I rang and woke an interstate colleague who had been Shirley's midwife for Lachlan's birth, and I knew she would be eager to know how the birth went. She was very sobered by my account and reassured me he was so lucky to have had the shoulder dystocia at home with a known midwife than with strangers in a hospital. She told me that two healthy baby boys had died as a result of shoulder dystocia in her local hospital that year. It was nice to have a friend and colleague reassure me so early in the morning. She said that it was a good time to have our talk, as she would be getting up soon to go for her early morning walk. I was so thankful she had been there to listen to me.

I snatched a few hours' restless sleep before getting back to Shirley and Alistair, and as we started on the next of what was to become many of our long talks, she told me that during her labour she had known she couldn't get her baby out herself. She was so tired, she confided, that she had just given up. She hoped she wasn't to blame for Alistair's arm being out of place during the labour.

Duncan and the boys also chatted many times during my visits over the next two weeks. We all came to realise that each of us had played a vital role in bringing Alistair into the world safely, but each time I visited during the following week I cringed when I saw what I had done to his little arm. I gradually came to terms with his temporary discomfort as I saw daily improvement.

Return of function in Alistair's damaged arm was mostly due to the continued attention and 'therapy' from his brothers. Each time Alistair woke for a feed, one of the boys would place his finger in the palm of his unresponsive hand, while at the same time talking to him and trying to stimulate his grasp reflex. The whole family let out a huge cheer the day they saw Alistair complete his first Moro reflex. The boys rang me at home to say they had taught him how to do it! Later, I saw for myself, as Alistair raised his damaged right arm together with his left. While driving home excitedly, I gave my belated victory cheer and made my usual gesture to any other driver who could see me.

Alistair Gough was weighed in at 4750 grams a few days after his birth. He responded well to the therapeutic care of his parents and brothers, and could move his right arm without apparent discomfort ten days later.

His right-hand grasp became stronger with the persistent stimulation provided by Lachlan and Callum, and within a few weeks he had a full range of movement. He received a clean bill of health from the consulting paediatrician who examined him when he was about a month old. The paediatrician congratulated us all on a job well done, and said he didn't need to see Alistair again.

Now when I hear the words 'shoulder dystocia' being bandied around at professional gatherings, I think of Alistair, and give thanks for being able to help him out.

A family affair

HELEN SANDNER

It wasn't an ordinary Saturday. My grandchildren – Alice, aged seven, and Rhen, five – had come to stay for a week of the school holidays. With breakfast over it was time to plan the morning – shopping and then a visit to my 92-year-old father. Alice and Rhen chose to come with Grandma, knowing that they would get to visit 'Pop Pop'.

Just before we left home, the phone rang. It was Sally, a midwife with whom I had arranged to back up for a planned homebirth.

Good news: her client, Sue, had started to labour. It was her first baby; labour had commenced around eight o'clock that morning and it was now 9.30 am. Nothing to worry about – Sally was available, and therefore there was no need for me to make special arrangements for the morning. Alec was home and could care for the girls if I was needed later on.

So, off to the shops. As we were tackling the dreaded supermarket shopping, my mobile phone rang. 'Hi, Helen? This is Brett,' said the voice on the other end. 'Sue is feeling pressure and would like a midwife with her,' he said. 'Sally is already on her way.'

Brett was concerned because Sally lived about an hour's drive from their home.

I thought to myself: This is Sue's first baby, and she hasn't been in labour that long. Maybe the baby is in a posterior position or the head is slightly deflexed. Maybe that's giving her a sense of pressure, and the need to push.

'Support her,' I suggested to Brett, 'and encourage her to rock and breathe through her contractions. If that doesn't help, it may be an idea for her to get down on all fours with her bottom in the air.' I left him with some more reassurances, and went back to the shopping.

We took far more time than I would usually want to spend in a supermarket, because Alice and Rhen were busy picking out treats to put in the trolley. We weren't quite done when the phone rang again.

'Hello again, Helen,' Brett said tensely. 'Sue's becoming very anxious.'

He told me that Sally hadn't yet arrived, but wasn't far away. My immediate thought was to check if the baby was low in the birth canal. I stood near the ice-cream freezer feeling self-conscious and trying to speak in a low voice.

'Can you feel inside Sally's vagina to see if you can touch the baby's head?' I whispered to Brett.

He checked and came back to the phone quickly. 'Yes!' he said, breathing fast. 'I can feel the baby's head. It's not far in!'

In the background, I heard a powerful pushing roar from Sue. It was the most wonderful sound that a midwife can hear, but not while she is standing in the middle of a supermarket!

'Brett, I'm on my way!' I yelled.

I quickly asked a couple of staff members to put my trolley aside. 'I'm needed at a birth – I'll be back!' I called, hardly registering their expressions of surprise.

'Quick, Alice and Rhen,' I said to the girls, grabbing their hands. 'We have to go to a birth!'

I buckled them up in the car and we were on our way. There was no time to take them home to be with their grandfather, so there was a quick lesson for them in the essentials of childbirth as I drove.

'Women having babies make noises, they feel pain which helps the baby to be born, but it's okay, so don't worry if you hear anything,' I reassured them. 'You won't be able to come into the room with me while the baby is being born, but you will be able to sit in another room. You'll need to be very quiet, okay?'

They both knew that they'd been born by Caesarian section, so I also had to explain that this baby would be born through Sue's vagina. Immediately, they wanted to know if my children had been born through my vagina!

Phew, no more time for questions! We pulled up in front of Sue and Brett's home. Leaving the girls to play on the front verandah, I ran into the house, to be greeted with the most amazing sight.

Sue was kneeling on all fours with Brett close beside

her. The baby's head had travelled well beyond the opening of her vagina. There was calm, and the most wonderful sense of 'oneness' between Sue and Brett. They were birthing their own baby. No doubt my presence was reassuring to them, but their strength and empowerment was amazing to see.

Sally rushed through the door not far behind me, but Brett and Sue were doing fine.

To see Brett cup his hands and then gently pass their baby to Sue was incredible. One day, I imagined, they would say to each other: *we did it ourselves.*

I watched Sue and Brett embracing and welcoming their baby with love, then went out to check on Alice and Rhen while Sally remained on hand. There was no need to tell the girls the baby had been born. They had heard the most wonderful first cry.

'Can we go now?' they asked.

I explained that I needed to stay a little longer because the placenta hadn't been born.

'How long will that be?' they asked.

'Anything from a few minutes to an hour or more,' I replied.

'Oh, no!' they shouted. Then Alice asked me curiously: 'What *is* the placenta?'

I explained.

'Well, what do they do with it?'

'The parents may like to bury the placenta in the garden and plant a tree on top of it,' I suggested, 'as a celebration of their baby's birth.'

Whatever I said appeared to become less and less acceptable to the children. They glanced at each other with expressions of distaste.

'There's nothing awful about our bodies,' I said. 'Bodies are beautiful, and the placenta is a very important and beautiful part of a mummy's body.'

I encouraged them to play outside for a little longer, then went back into the house to find that Sue had birthed her placenta. I sat quietly for a moment or two, embracing the intimate and joyful atmosphere of birth as I watched Sue and Brett getting to know their baby. Then I said goodbye and left them to enjoy their time together. I gathered up the children and we returned to collect our shopping trolley and then to visit 'Pop Pop'.

My sense of joy was intense – to have been present for such a wonderful birth, and for Alice and Rhen to have experienced a baby's birth at home, was more than I could have hoped for. I can only hope that in the future, if and when their time comes, they will have the options and the choice to birth their babies wherever they wish.

A SHOULDER to CRY ON

People don't know what we do

MAREE EGGLESTON

My patient – or client, as we have now been told to call them – relaxes into sleep as the epidural takes effect. The infusion pump ticks reassuringly. Observations remain normal. The Syntocinon drip is set at 40 millilitres per hour sustaining two- to three-minutely contractions, and the CTG graphs a healthy foetal heart rate. The mother-to-be nods when I wake her to explain the necessity for a urinary catheter; she is dozing again when I insert it. Urine the colour of lemon cordial rushes into the drainage bag. A vaginal examination reveals that the cervix is 6 centimetres dilated. Good, we're getting there. A baby should be in the cot before the end of the shift. My charts are all up to date. I'll get a meal break today.

'I'm going to grab some lunch,' I say to the father. 'If

you're worried about anything, ring the buzzer and I'll come back.'

'I will.' He smiles. 'Thank God for epidurals.'

I leave the delivery suite for the first time in hours. The main corridor is a mess. You could be excused for thinking a bloody battle has just been waged there. Delivery trolleys line the walls waiting their turn to be stripped and cleaned. Judging by the splashing, banging and crashing coming from the pan room, they'll be there a while. A lot happened out here while I was occupied in my room. On my way to the tearoom I have to pick a path through an obstacle course of trolleys, cots and linen skips.

Gabi pokes her head around the bathroom door. 'Have you got a minute?'

'I was about to eat my lunch.'

'It won't take long.'

'Sure.' I try not to sound reluctant. My salad sandwich will have to wait.

The previous occupant to languish in the bath must have used the oil burner because a hint of lavender hovers. Gabi closes the door. The bath, a handbasin and three spare cots fill the room.

'What's up?' I ask.

'Sorry, but I can't do this on my own.' Gabi nods towards one of the cots. A tiny bump under the white cotton blanket says it all.

'A 23-weeker,' says Gabi. 'I've washed and dressed her. Now I'm doing the album for the parents.' She pulls a booklet from the shelf under the cot and opens it to the first page. The Polaroid snapshot silently shrieks of death; face waxen, eyes sealed, lips black. Underneath, a few strands of dark hair held fast by sticky tape. Precise lettering in blue texta spells out a name, Lilly, and the date and time of her birth.

'She's been dead a while. At least 24 hours before the delivery. So there's a bit of skin slip. I can't get the hand- and footprints without doing some damage. It'll be easier if there are two of us.'

I nod.

We stand on either side of the cot. Gabi peels back the blanket from the still, pale form that is Lilly. The sea-green dress swims around her. Embroidered rosebuds encircle her neck and dot the puffed sleeves. I can't stop my fingers from cupping her tiny head and my thumb from stroking her chilled brow. In unison, Gabi and I exhale a sighing breath. 'Let's do it.'

Fingers edge beneath Lilly's wrist and I raise her spindly arm. Gabi slips the ink-pad under a fragile, floppy hand. I hold my breath and press the palm on to ink the colour of a fresh bruise. And one by one, each tiny finger and the thumb. I sense the skin give and hesitate. But no harm is done, and when Gabi holds the album open, a blank page feels an inky hand.

Gabi nods. 'Not bad. Now for the foot.'

My hand cradles a skeletal leg around the calf. As the heel loses contact with the mattress, skin frees from muscle at the ankle and slides up to gather around the knee like a silk sleeve. Exposed flesh, deep purple, glistens with decomposition.

Our combined gasp stabs into the silence.

'Don't worry,' whispers Gabi. 'Just do the best you can.'

I lean further into the cot and ease the tube of skin

back down to the ankle and carefully, very carefully, hold it in place. The foot, and each bud that is a toe, brush the ink-pad, and as fleetingly as a butterfly kiss, I let it touch the paper.

The prints rest side by side. Faint, insubstantial, smudged, but clearly a foot and a hand.

Gabi is silent, staring.

'What's wrong? Do you think I could have done a better job?'

'No. It's not that. The prints have turned out better than I thought they would.'

'What, then?'

'I was thinking. Look at us. Look at what we just did. You should have seen your face. You concentrated so hard, were so careful.' Gabi shakes her head slowly. 'People don't know what we do.'

'Gabi, most of the time, *we* don't know what we do.'

'You're probably right. But anyway, thanks for the help. Sorry I had to ask.'

'I didn't mind. In a way, it's a privilege.'

'I know what you mean. Grab a break before you're needed.'

I shovel down lunch and return to my patient/client and her partner. Two hours later, I leave the delivery suite to head home with the angry bellowing of a 3915-gram baby girl drumming in my ears.

A birth story written with regret

ANNIE SPRAGUE

The 'birth plan' meeting at 36 weeks gestation is my opportunity to be together with you and your family and to talk over any 'housekeeping' tasks before the big day.

I arrive and am invited into your space. We walk around the house and admire the newly set-up baby's crib. We talk about the preparations you have made, and smile as we look at your two boys eagerly awaiting this new spirit. I thought you seemed so reserved and quiet tonight. That funny viral infection you have had over the last couple of weeks has left you with a nagging cough.

'You'll have to go to the doctor's tomorrow and get something done about that cough,' I say.

'Yes,' you agree. 'I'm sure the baby is sick of hearing me cough.'

We move into the lounge room so that I can feel your tummy and listen to the baby's heart. Your eldest son's hands follow my hands across your tummy and together we trace the shape of the baby inside. The baby is lying in a good position with the head deep inside the pelvis. I take out my sonicaid as we chat and I listen for the babe's heartbeat.

I can't hear anything.

My stomach rolls and I feel sick. I try a different spot. 'Maybe,' I say to the four pairs of watching eyes, 'the baby is a bit posterior and we'll hear the heartbeat further out on the flank.'

Still no sound.

All I can hear is the rock music coming through the wall from the next-door neighbours'. I comment that I hope they don't play music that loud while you are in labour, as I frantically try to find the heartbeat.

I think that I must have made a mistake with my abdominal palpation, and that maybe the baby is breech. I start to listen all over your belly. Still no heartbeat.

You are all looking at me and the room is so quiet. Your youngest son, who is used to me listening and feeling, is now touching your tummy and saying 'Baby'.

I have to speak up and say to you that I cannot hear anything, and you very calmly look me in the eye and say that you think your baby has died.

You say that you have felt no movements since yesterday, or maybe the day before, but you weren't overly worried as the same thing happened during your last pregnancy, when you went rushing off to the hospital for a CTG and everything was okay.

I ask your partner to get you a glass of iced water. 'We can't be sure yet,' I say, but my stomach is sick with worry.

It's just so awful. I try to get a response by prodding the baby and giving you the water to drink, but still there's nothing.

We discuss what to do next. I ring the hospital and speak to the obstetric registrar, to let her know what has happened. We ring for someone to come and mind your youngest child while we all sit, stunned, but unable to give up hope.

My mind is racing back to all our previous antenatal visits and I wonder if I have missed something.

It's freezing cold and dark when we leave to drive to the hospital. The overwhelming tiredness I felt earlier and the headache from lack of sleep have miraculously disappeared. I offer to take your eldest son with me in my car, as much for his company on the drive to the hospital as well as to give you and your partner some privacy.

We present ourselves to the Emergency department and together we walk up to the strange and slightly alien environment of the labour ward. The staff we meet are all lovely to us. The midwife brings in the CTG machine so that we can listen for the baby.

Nothing.

Yes, there *is* something. But when I hold your hand I realise that the 'beat' is only your racing pulse. The midwife thought it might have been the baby's heartbeat, but you and I look at each other and say that no, the baby's heart didn't sound like that. We both knew how his heart sounded when you came to my house for antenatal visits.

We page the doctor to come, and even though you don't really want to have an ultrasound you both agree that it's the only thing we can really do to know for certain.

We see the baby, his small hands lying so still, cradling his head. We see the chest cavity and the heart, but there is no sign of life. I try not to cry, but the tears start to flow down my cheeks as my hand rests on your son's shoulder. You are so calm. It's still too unreal for it all to sink in.

I leave the room to go and make a cup of tea. Anything to stop me sobbing out loud.

You agree to have some blood and cervical swabs taken, even though you know that they might not give us any explanation to why this spirit has left so suddenly.

Your partner is so sad; I wish I could just take his pain away. Your son is so strong and fatalistic, as the young often are. It's good for me, to see him strong for you.

You just want to give birth to your baby. You tell the hospital staff and me that you would like to birth at home, as we planned. We are advised by the staff that they want you to 'deliver in hospital, as she might haemorrhage'.

You can't make a decision straight away and tell the staff you need to go home and digest what has happened. We leave the hospital just before midnight, each of us in our own state of shock, with the plan to return in the morning for induction with prostaglandin gel.

I wonder why I became a midwife, and why I am doing this job. A couple of days on the checkout counter at Coles supermarket doesn't sound half-bad. The weather is bitterly cold with a strong westerly wind blowing. It seems appropriate.

In the morning, you return to the hospital and have the gel inserted. According to the hospital staff, your cervix isn't very favourable and you might need more than one dose.

I feel very strongly that you will labour overnight, but tell you that you might also sleep all night. We 'check in' by phone before I go to bed, but already your body is subtly undergoing changes with some very strong uterine actions.

Twelve-fifteen in the early hours of the morning.

'This is it,' your partner says into the phone, and I am already out of my warm bed and into a clear but cold and starry night. I have packed my resuscitation gear, as requested by you and agreed by me. There is never any certainty in life.

I take ten minutes at that hour to arrive at your home. As I walk into the softly lit room that you have set up to birth in, I'm greeted by a look of immense satisfaction and power as you smile at me from the birth pool with your son cradled in your arms. It is so beautiful. I look at the faces of your children supporting you and welcoming their new brother who is stillborn.

That word isn't so bad now that I can see it in the true context of its meaning. He is so still and looks so very much at peace. His body, though small, is perfect, with no obvious sign as to why he chose to leave before we knew him.

I feel really proud for you to have given birth to him at home in the water as planned, and to be invited by you both to share such an unforgettable moment.

Later on that day, I start a jigsaw puzzle with my children, and it is so appropriate as an analogy for life. The pieces are all laid out. There is no obvious pattern and yet slowly, we begin to make sense of the pieces.

They fit, where once there was only doubt and confusion.

The woman in this story became pregnant within two years of losing her baby and had a beautiful baby girl at home. The circle was completed.

Filling up

SHONA DAVIDSON

We were sitting in the back of the ambulance at the petrol station filling up with fuel when it happened. A petrol station, of all places . . .

The day had begun like any other. Arrived at work, made a coffee, got handover from the previous shift, checked the equipment, and was sitting down to catch up with some paperwork when the call came in.

It was a request from a rural hospital to retrieve a baby with heart disease diagnosed at birth. Her condition was deteriorating. The baby, who was by now a couple of months old, was having difficulty breathing. So off we set in our ambulance, just like any other retrieval. En route, the doctor, Frank, and I chatted through the various scenarios we could find, discussed our 'plan of attack', and calculated the dosage of drugs we may potentially use, before we settled back to watch the scenery pass. However, although you may look relaxed, enjoying the countryside even, your mind is constantly ticking over. *Is the cot plugged in? Did I take the extra drugs with me? Is the mobile switched on . . .*

Very relieved-looking staff greeted us when we arrived at the referring hospital – an indicator that perhaps the baby's condition had deteriorated. This was confirmed when we entered the special care nursery. The baby, Emily, was in severe respiratory distress. After introductions to Emily's parents, we quickly wheeled in our equipment and I attached Emily to our monitoring system, jotted down her heart and respiratory rate, blood pressure, and so on, while doing a quick assessment at the same time. Frank busied himself explaining to the family what we were doing, and the treatment needed. Their consent obtained, we prepared Emily. She needed a breathing tube, and this was soon inserted and attached to our ventilator.

Emily was very sick and it took us some time to get her stabilised enough for transfer. Once she was settled into our transport cot, we left her alone with her family for a few precious minutes.

Mum, Dad and older sister all gave her a kiss through their tears. We'd explained that she was critically ill, and had offered for one of her parents to travel with her in the ambulance. They declined the offer, saying they would prefer to travel to the city together, '. . . knowing that Emily was in good hands'. Our hands.

With a final goodbye, we loaded everything into the back of the ambulance. After an equipment check, baby check and phone call to base informing them of Emily's condition, we were off.

'Call it nurse's intuition or whatever, but I'm not feeling quite right about this transfer,' I confided to Frank.

'Nurse's intuition,' he scoffed, before admitting he wasn't feeling too comfortable either.

We watched the baby like a cat watches a mouse . . . waiting for the wrong move. The journey, however, was going smoothly. Emily's condition, while critical, remained stable.

'Gotta stop for some diesel, folks. Sorry, but I thought we'd have enough to get us back,' came a voice from up front.

'Okay, but hurry,' I replied, a little annoyed.

'Couldn't you have done that before we left the hospital?' I thought privately, which was most ungracious as the ambulance officer had been very busy helping us to stabilise Emily.

And that was when it happened.

The ambo was outside filling the tanks, when the monitor suddenly showed an irregularity in Emily's heart rate. I opened the cot doors to check her, and it happened again. This time, however, the heart rate didn't spontaneously revert to normal, but continued to deteriorate.

'Starting compressions,' said the doctor, as I commenced hand-ventilating the baby.

'Air entry clear,' I told the doctor.

'Well, a blocked breathing tube's not the problem,' I thought.

'Get the office on the speaker-phone,' I yelled to the ambulance officer outside the car, 'and get the drug box opened!'

Hearing the urgency in my voice, he immediately came to help us.

We had given some emergency drugs with no effect when the senior medical officer back at the base came on the speaker-phone. We quickly updated him on what had happened and what we had done.

'Give more adrenalin,' he instructed.

'Adrenalin fourth dose going in,' replied the doctor, as he pushed the drug. We waited, watching for what was beginning to seem like an eternity . . .

'No effect, recommencing CPR.'

'Give another adrenalin.'

'Give bicarb.'

'Give some calcium.'

The instructions kept coming from the voice back at base. It remained calm and supportive as we kept them updated with the result. Nothing was having any effect.

Finally, after 40 minutes of active resuscitation with no result, the voice spoke again. 'Okay, stop what you are doing and assess the baby.'

'No spontaneous resps, no cardiac output, pupils fixed and dilated.'

There was a pause. 'Okay, guys. You have tried very hard, but you must stop now, do you understand?'

There was a terrible silence. We all looked at each other.

'Are you alright?' I asked the doctor, realising the futility of carrying on.

He nodded.

'Yes,' I told base.

'Oh, dear. Well, then, record the time of death. Keep going to your receiving hospital. We'll inform them of what's happened and we'll contact the parents for you. Will you all be okay?'

There was a long silence before we could reply.

With heavy hearts, we tidied the usual detritus that follows a resuscitation. Then I remembered where we were.

'God, a bloody petrol station!' I thought. We switched off the monitor, and I gently wrapped Emily in a blanket.

'I'm sorry, little one,' I said to her as I tied the safety harness around her. 'Rest in peace.'

I closed the transport cot lid and pulled the covers over, and we resumed our journey to the city. We were all very quiet, lost in our own thoughts. Did we miss something? Was there more we could have done? Did we pull out too early?

The doctor and I checked and re-checked our notes of the whole transfer – it didn't seem like we had missed something. We tried to convince each other that we'd done all we could, but neither of us succeeded. Then the voice from the overhead speaker interrupted our thoughts.

'We can't trace the parents. They've left the referring hospital, are not at home and their mobile is off. We'll keep trying. Just keep on to the receiving hospital. They might be waiting for you there.'

'Oh, God. We still have to speak to the parents,' I thought.

This had completely escaped my thoughts. There is nothing more haunting than the cry a mother makes when you tell her that her baby has died. It's a sound like no other. One you really should never have to hear. And here we were, sitting in the back of our ambulance, with a baby we had tried hard to save, and failed, and her parents still didn't know.

The doctor, the ambo and I really supported each other on the return journey home. With all that we had just been through, and knowing what was to come, an unspoken bond formed.

When we arrived back in the city, the parents still hadn't arrived, and they still hadn't been contacted. We must have looked more shell-shocked than we realised. The receiving hospital staff gently took Emily from us and steered us into their tearoom, where they gave us hot, sweet tea. The inane drivel from the television couldn't distract us from our thoughts. We were gutted. Truly gutted.

When a patient whose life you have been entrusted with dies, you constantly question your skills, your knowledge, your practice. It's a cycle that goes around and around in your head. Sometimes there's resolution, but more often there's not. You want to cry, you feel you should, but you're frightened to. You know that the years of accumulated grief will surge to the fore like a tidal wave and you'll drown. So, you sit there. Staring at nothing.

We waited for quite some time for the parents to arrive, but still they didn't show. Meanwhile, another referral call had come in. We had to get back to the office and re-stock and get back out on the road. It was time to put on yet another happy face, bury the grief, hope it could be dealt with another day.

We had to leave Emily. We never got the chance to explain to her parents what had happened. To say how hard we had tried to save their baby. To say how very sorry we were for their loss.

Not just a day job

GENEVIEVE LILLEY

Recently a card arrived at the birth centre where I work. It was from a woman who had given birth to her second child, a daughter she had named Sharney, a year earlier, with me as her midwife. Already one year ago, I thought . . . .

The last time I saw the woman, Lynne, I hadn't immediately recognised her, which was odd. I had thought a lot about the birth and the events that had followed, and cried many tears during that time – it was a birth I'll never forget. It was one of the most memorable shifts I have worked as a midwife, where I was in the presence of love, struggle, raw vulnerability, joyous achievement, fear, grief, shock and extraordinary bravery.

It was a busy night in the birth centre, and I was working with one other midwife called Aileen. There were two or three women in labour with their partners, including Lynne and her husband Wayne.

Lynne seemed a very reserved sort of person, and although she was having some strong contractions, she didn't appear distressed by them. Wayne had been at work since early that morning and looked really exhausted. I suggested he may need a 'power nap' before Lynne's labour progressed any further. Lynne and Wayne were left largely to themselves for the next hour or two, while Aileen and I attended to the other women in the centre.

At one stage, Lynne came out to ask for some towels, as she wanted to go into the shower for a while. She still didn't seem distressed by the contractions and I took this as a sign that she wasn't yet in established labour. With hindsight, which is always a wonderful thing in childbirth, this was probably a hasty judgment based on her reserve and my preoccupation with the more pressing demands of the other women at that time. As it turned out, she was labouring well and reappeared not too much later to tell me she was feeling an urge to push when she had a contraction. We went back into her room, woke Wayne, and prepared for the birth.

Aileen came in to help as the baby's arrival came closer. Lynne knelt on a mat next to the bed to give birth. Everything went smoothly, and a big healthy baby was soon born and quickly made some angry-sounding crying noises. I remember Wayne, who had been struggling with fatigue not long earlier, looking up at Lynne and saying through tears of joy: 'It's a little girl! A little girl!'

Lynne cuddled her new daughter close to her body. The baby's cries stayed irregular, but otherwise she looked fine – her colour was good, her heart was beating strongly, and she was flexing her arms and legs. After a few minutes, however, her breathing was still irregular and we decided that Aileen should take her out to the resuscitation cot to assess her more thoroughly. I wasn't particularly worried about her – it seemed like a precaution more than anything else. She was a lovely healthy baby, with a normal heart rate, good colour and muscle tone, and she had cried immediately after she was born. What could go wrong?

I stayed with Lynne to deliver the placenta. When I ducked out of the room shortly afterwards to get something, I saw that Aileen had called a doctor who was examining the baby. Everything seemed calm. Back in the labour room, Wayne was clearly getting worried, and I think at that time I suggested he go out and stay with the baby. I expected him to bring her back in shortly so that she could breastfeed.

A few minutes later, when I went out again, the situation had changed dramatically. A crowd of doctors and intensive care nurses was gathered around the baby – obviously someone had called the emergency code and I hadn't heard it from inside the labour room. I could see that the suction tubing had a lot of blood in it. Everyone was focused intently on the resuscitation. I was horrified to see Wayne sitting at the nurses' station alone, his head in his hands. The terrible possibility that the baby was dying suddenly occurred to me.

I had seen an unsuccessful resuscitation on a stillborn baby once before, and a familiar sensation of dread started to creep up on me. I couldn't understand what had happened – there had been nothing wrong with *this* baby. Where had all that blood come from? Newborn babies don't bleed. At least, they're not supposed to.

Eventually the baby was taken to the neonatal intensive care unit (NICU), and one of the doctors came in to explain what had happened. I really don't remember what he said, but the message was bleak: *bleeding in the lungs . . . unstable . . . we'll call you when we have any news*. He was in a hurry to follow the baby to the nursery.

The next few hours passed in a blur. I went about doing the normal things that I would be doing anyway – cleaning up, checking Lynne's blood pressure – but I felt like an automaton, performing actions that had lost their usual significance in the sudden uprooting of normal priorities. Lynne remained calm, unreadable, while she waited for news of her baby. They had called her Sharney.

It was a couple of hours before we were called. I negotiated my way through all the cots and machines with Lynne in a wheelchair towards the far end of the intensive care nursery. Again, there was a crowd gathered around the baby, except now most of them were hanging back waiting to see if their work of the last few hours was paying off.

In spite of all the attention from all those experts with all their accumulated experience, and all that high-tech equipment, the baby now looked terrible (though it was precisely because of all that stuff that she was still alive at all).

Sharney was attached via a breathing tube to a respirator called an oscillator, which pumps oxygen into the lungs rapidly and shallowly, several times per second. It caused her body to jerk with each in/out flow of oxygen. Even with this mechanical assistance, she was mottled blue and purple all over. Occasionally she lifted an arm, and seemed to breathe against the rhythm of the oscillator. This looked good to me – from the colour of her, you wouldn't have thought she could do anything. Two nurses were busy securing tubes and monitor wires. Everyone was grim-faced.

An older doctor, the senior paediatrician, talked to Lynne and Wayne. He didn't say anything promising. They had just spent a couple of hours trying to correct complications from oxygen deprivation, which had occurred after a bleed into the lungs. They weren't sure why it had happened; they didn't know how things were going to go. Her condition, as I recall, was described as 'grave'.

Lynne asked for a photo to be taken of herself, Wayne and Sharney, and one of the nurses complied. Lynne remained inscrutable. Her composure struck me as extraordinary – it was as if some protective instinct came into play that allowed her to focus on her baby without giving in to fear.

Standing behind them, I was feeling anything but composed. Tears welled in my eyes. Memories of that other baby that had died gripped me, and I felt devastated by the sight of the blue and purple baby on the cot struggling to breathe and move, and by the thought of what might lie ahead for these parents.

Just then the day supervisor, Beverley, who does a hospital round at 6.30 every morning, called to say I had to return to the birth centre straightaway. I left Lynne and Wayne in the nursery, and hurried off.

The next days and weeks were very difficult. I went home that day believing that Sharney would die, an unbearable thought. I cried and cried. I was rostered off for several days and I couldn't bring myself to ring up to hear the news. I wanted to avoid the grief that I could feel lurking whenever I thought about the possibility.

It may seem strange to feel such grief for people I didn't even know very well, but it seems to be part of the equation of midwifery – you get to share the joy of birth, but when things go wrong you also share the grief. Most of the time, even when it's a difficult labour, the birth heralds the end of the pain and distress of labour and brings joy and wonderment. When things go wrong and a baby is sick or dies, part of the joy and euphoria that you feel whenever a well baby is born after that is actually relief.

Eventually, one of my colleagues called to let me know that Sharney was still alive. She had suffered oxygen deprivation and had cerebral oedema as a result, but her condition had improved. Although the cerebral oedema had seen her fitting and potentially suffering permanent brain damage, she was by then no longer 'gravely' ill.

When I returned to work, I was eager to visit the nursery to see her. However, when I approached the attending nurse, she abruptly and immediately told me that I 'should have called the code sooner'. I was later flummoxed by her insensitivity, and by the fact that she had no interest in knowing about what actually happened at the time. People in hospitals can be very quick to point the finger when things go wrong, and although I felt confident about my judgment at the time, it sent me into a tailspin of self-recrimination and endless 'what ifs'.

In the second week after Sharney's birth, while we were waiting for an MRI to assess her brain function, I was plagued with thoughts of how her and her family's life might be affected if she had severe brain damage. I wondered if I could have done something to alter the course of events. Ask any midwife how that feels – and, in the words of one of my colleagues, some days you wonder why you don't just get a job in a pie shop.

And then something happens to remind you of why you don't. On the night Sharney was born, when I was called back to the birth centre from the nursery, I had wiped the tears from my eyes and invoked the old nursing power of emotional repression in the face of multiple and pressing tasks.

I wasn't sure what I was going to find, but when Beverley summons you, you know it's probably something important. In this instance, she had found one of our women in the bath and pretty close to giving birth, without a midwife in sight. They were on the way back to her room when I returned.

It was a bit of a struggle getting her on to the bed – it's a terrible time to be moving, when the baby's head is so low down – you really have to cajole every tiny movement out of a woman when she's pushing, and by the time I got there she was pushing really hard.

She and her partner were a lovely starry-eyed young couple – the sort of people who seem always to be smiling and happy, and full of youthful exuberance. Although it was her first baby, her labour had been quick and she had coped well, so they were both brimming with positive energy. She managed to get on to all fours on the bed and her boyfriend was encouraging her excitedly. He peered down behind her and saw the baby's head coming down as she pushed.

'I can see the head, hon! I can see the baby's head!' He was as excited as a kid in a lolly shop. Somehow she managed to respond in kind, even though she was clearly in a lot of pain at that stage: 'Can you, hon?'

She was pushing with great determination, but her sunny disposition was still evident. I can't remember her name, or her partner's name, and I wouldn't recognise her if I saw her now. But I remember her strength and power and the love that flowed so freely between them. The woman screamed long and loud during the birth, but as soon as their baby girl was born, she cried – a healthy cry! Such regular, normal-sounding crying! What relief! And then they were both laughing ecstatically and so happy and filled with pure joy and exuberance that I *almost* forgot where I had been only half an hour earlier . . .

And as for Lynne and Wayne? It was a long and difficult journey for them, too, and one that makes my own pale into insignificance. But the story of Sharney's illness and rather miraculous recovery is theirs to tell, and incidentally, one that Lynne hopes to one day make into a storyboard to add to the others that line the corridors of the NICU. But I will give the ending away here, by telling you what Lynne wrote in that card she sent us on the occasion of Sharney's first birthday: 'Sharney is doing fantastic – she is better than perfect! She has been walking for about a month now and is going great guns.'

Ask any midwife – that's why I won't be taking a job in a pie shop.

Keeping time

KATE FIELD

'What a beautiful old watch; a Waltham, isn't it?' said Ruth, carefully lowering her pregnant form on to the narrow triage bed. She was a regular outpatient having frequent monitoring for a small baby.

I couldn't remember how long I'd had the watch. My husband arrived home with it one day from the auctions. The creamy enamel face and soft gold surrounds gleamed back at me under the stark fluorescent lights.

'It *is* a nice watch,' I agreed, checking Ruth's pulse and watching the gold hand sweep around.

The watch was such an integral part of midwifery practice, sometimes a curse though, determining how much longer a woman would be 'allowed' to labour, or to push.

I listened to Ruth's baby, counting the steady rhythm, smiling with the mother at the reassuring beat.

Sometimes, though, the reassuring sound is absent. Another pregnant woman, Claire, rang during the afternoon shift, worried that her baby hadn't moved all day. Not an uncommon concern, but always cause for a visit to the hospital. I skimmed through her history while awaiting her arrival. Claire was expecting her third child the following week and had a history of two quick births. Her sons were three and two years old.

She arrived looking concerned, but not distraught. Straight dark hair framed her open, friendly face.

'Hi, I'm Kate. I spoke to you on the phone,' I said.

'Dan's down parking the car. He won't be long.' She positioned herself on the triage couch and looked at the CTG monitor in the corner.

'That's for monitoring the baby's heart,' I explained, wheeling it closer.

'I know,' she said, anxiety in her dark eyes. She had one of those neat pregnant bellies, like a basketball. The type that magazine covers display.

'It's probably just having a deep sleep. They usually kick like mad when we put the monitor on.' Empty platitudes given the possible circumstances, I thought. But how many women come in with reduced movements and everything's fine?

'Actually, I've felt sick the last couple of days, like I'm coming down with something,' she reflected.

Claire's husband burst in the door. 'Had trouble parking! God, your belly looks like it's shrunk, when you lie down like that.'

And that was when I knew without a doubt I wouldn't hear a foetal heart. This wasn't going to be one of those quiet babies that squirmed into activity with prompting.

Claire's abdomen felt cool, the stillness palpable. I felt around for the baby's position, willing it to kick in response. The fundal height was small for gestation.

I squeezed the gel on to the transducer and watched Claire as I slid the piece from one side of her abdomen to the other, and back again. Inert silence. She stared at the monitor, waiting for the sound of galloping hoof beats. A tear slid down her cheek. She knew as well.

What do you say?

I glanced down at my watch; there would still be a sonographer in ultrasound.

'I'm sorry, I can't pick it up with this. I'll just ring the doctor. I'll be right back. Don't think the worst.'

I grasped her hand and felt her desperate fear. I pulled a chair over for Dan to sit by Claire. He hadn't said a word.

The registrar arrived promptly, had a brief listen and booked an urgent ultrasound.

I sat with Claire, and Dan made some calls.

'What happens now? I'm so scared,' she whispered.

'I know. We'll go down to ultrasound with the doctor and take it from there.'

'They said it was a girl, the last time I had a scan. I really wanted a girl.' The tears streamed relentlessly.

'Claire, just wait for the ultrasound.' She gripped my hand.

So, downstairs we went with a faint glimmer of hope. The black screen dominated the room as once again Claire's belly was covered in gel. The sonographer chased the images around, but all we could hear was the soft ticking of my watch. The form gradually evolved: head, body, limbs. Motionless, suspended in timeless space, the tiny heart rigid.

'I'm very sorry, the baby has died,' said the sonographer, matter-of-factly.

'Oh God, no,' moaned Claire. 'Oh, Dan, Dan.'

Their raw pain filled the cubicle as they held each other. I blinked back tears.

'How did it happen?' choked Dan.

The registrar shook her head. 'We'll talk upstairs. I'm very sorry. This is a very sad thing.'

We returned to the ward, Claire sobbing quietly.

'I'm so sorry,' I said simply.

'But how long has it been like that?' gulped Claire. 'When did it happen?'

'I don't know. I guess we'll have a better idea after . . . after it's born.'

The time of birth of this baby would be preceded by an unknown time of death.

The registrar sat on the bed and explained the options and expected outcomes. Claire chose to go home that night after some prostaglandin gel and would return in the morning.

She hugged me fiercely and we wept together. The next day she would give birth to her stillborn baby girl, Anna, who was bathed and cuddled and dressed, her perfect footprints placed in a book.

Claire and Dan went home to a silent nursery.

Some people say that time heals.

I slipped my watch off and felt it warm in my hand before laying it on the bedside table, the gold hands sweeping around.

AFTER the BIRTH

Crossing cultures

SANDRA LINKLATER

By the time I'd walked up the third flight of stairs with the bag containing the baby scales my heart was beating faster than a rock star playing a drum solo. Sweat was dribbling down the side of my neck. My new cotton blouse clung to my body as if I had worn it for Sydney's City to Surf fun run.

It was spring, a time of the year when a slight sea breeze fans the sunny days in the suburb where I work. On a normal day, two or three mothers would be walking together and the park on the corner would be full of children. But today was one of those days where the temperature had suddenly hit 35 degrees after a week of being in the low twenties.

As I stopped to catch my breath and have a drink from my water bottle, I wondered how parents coped, living in a high-rise unit where the living space was restricted to three or four rooms. Without lifts, just going out for the day would take enormous effort.

The front door to the unit block was chocked open with a piece of wood. The stairwell was dark and smelled of cats. The windows rattled slightly as a train passed by on the railway track next to the building. Just down the street a new block of units was being built. The noise from the construction site reminded me of a news report I had seen the night before on the war in Iraq.

I was looking for Unit 21. The name of the client was Lucy Wong. Lucy had delivered a healthy boy that morning at the local hospital. She had been discharged soon after because she didn't have a Medicare card. The discharge nurse had rung the child and family health centre where I worked to ask if I could do a follow-up home visit the same day.

I had rung Lucy one hour later and been greeted by a young woman speaking Mandarin. She hung up on me very rapidly when I said 'English'. I spent another half-hour on the phone trying to arrange for a Mandarin interpreter to meet me at her address. I failed; no interpreters were available until the following week.

Two more hours went by before I contacted Lucy again with the help of the telephone interpreter service and set up an appointment for that afternoon. The conversation had been tedious and at one point the telephone interpreter had asked: 'Is she alright? She sounds a bit vague.'

As I raised my hand to knock on the door of Unit 21 I heard a muffled sound on the other side, then raised voices. I stood there for a few minutes wondering if I should leave or ring one of my colleagues for support. While I was making my decision the door opened and a petite Chinese woman with wide dark eyes that barely made contact with mine appeared.

Her thin lips parted in a smile that showed uneven yellow teeth. She lowered her gaze to the floor. Her long black hair was neatly brushed behind her ears and she was dressed in clean pink flannelette pyjamas, over which she wore a heavy grey overcoat. A toddler rested on her right hip snuggled into her chest; from behind her, another little face peeked out. The little girl looked to be about five years old. Her floral dress came down to her ankles.

Seeing pairs of shoes lined neatly up against the wall, I took my cue, removed my shoes and walked barefoot straight into the lounge/dining room where toys were scattered over the floor. The windows were closed with the curtains drawn. In one corner of the room, on the only visible table, was a computer. In the opposite corner, close to the front door, stood a Buddha, with offerings of flowers. There was one chair and a single, two-seater brown couch, decorated with a half-eaten packet of Smith's chips.

As I moved further into the room I could see the kitchen. There was no fridge. A half empty bottle of Coke stood on a green laminated benchtop, next to a handful of wilted vegetables. There was one window above the sink. It looked out on to a brick wall.

Lucy started to walk towards a closed door off the lounge room.

'Baby?' I asked. As her hand reached for the door handle, two more children between the ages of eight and eleven ran out of the room. I looked at the referral letter that had been faxed to me by the discharge nurse; it said there was only one child. So far I had counted four children in this one-bedroom unit.

Lucy reached down towards a bare double bed that occupied the centre of the room, and picked up a bundle swaddled in a woollen shawl, complete with an oversized bonnet on the small head. An electric heater was on next to the bed, and the sun streamed off the closed pink venetian blinds. I couldn't contain my impatience. 'Too hot!' I cried. 'Too hot.'

I began to pull off the baby's bonnet as Lucy lowered the child to the bed. Just then, one of the children came back into the room, climbed on to the bed and started to unwrap the baby. I removed the child's hands, muttering 'I'll do it'. The baby's thick black hair was glued to his scalp from moisture. The sleeves of the nightgown were pinned down so that he couldn't move his arms. His hands were covered with mittens. Without looking up at the faces that stared at me, I unpinned his arms. I was struggling to contain my anger. I knew, of course, that it was a Chinese tradition to keep a new baby warm, but this was excessive.

'Baby's name?' I asked dully.

'Peeper,' came the reply.

'Peter.'

'*Wey.* Yes.'

For the next hour, as I examined the baby, Lucy answered my questions and gesticulations 'wey', while the beeping sounds of a computer game could be heard in the background. When Peter began to cry, Lucy picked him up and nuzzled him to her breast. Her face was serene as she stroked his head and cooed to him in Mandarin.

As I was leaving the unit, my nursing instinct kicked in. I could see that Lucy loved her baby, but there was something wrong. I spent the following two days discussing my anxiety about Lucy with my colleagues and asking myself the same questions. Were all the children Lucy's? Did she have a partner? Why weren't the children in school?

A week later I was again knocking on the door of Unit 21, this time accompanied by a Mandarin interpreter. I was impatient to learn answers to my questions. The eldest child opened the door carrying Peter. He looked so peaceful I mistook him for a doll, but he wore no bonnet or wrap. One hand rested against his face, the other fell limply towards the floor.

As we settled ourselves on the couch, I noticed that the only thing that had changed in a week was the disappearance of the Coke bottle. I tried hard to keep my concerns hidden from Lucy and the interpreter.

'Lucy, where is your partner, the father of your children?'

Lucy didn't answer. Instead she reached into the pocket of her grey overcoat and pulled out a handful of documents. Some were in Mandarin, some in English. The room was unusually quiet as the four children huddled around Lucy's legs.

As I looked through the documents, the interpreter started chatting to Lucy in Mandarin, then looked towards me. 'I told her not to be frightened,' she said.

Nodding, I continued examining the papers. There were two Australian documents: a divorce certificate and a marriage certificate. Hesitantly, Lucy began to speak. At times the interpreter had difficulty translating.

Lucy showed no emotion as she talked of China's one child policy, the abortion she had to have. When she became pregnant for a third time, her husband had moved her through Hong Kong to Malaysia. Lucy had feared having another abortion, so with each successive pregnancy they had moved closer to Australia.

Here her husband had divorced her, after paying an Australian man to marry her. After Lucy had fallen pregnant, she never saw the Australian again. Now her Chinese husband had moved back in with Lucy and their children, but his visa had run out a week before Peter was born and he had been forced to return to China. Lucy believed that once she received permanent residency, her family could be reunited. In the meantime she was receiving money from China. The children had been doing the shopping and caring for each other, while Lucy struggled to live within the confines of Chinese tradition that forbade her to go out or do anything for 40 days following the birth of a baby except care for herself and her newborn child.

During the following weeks I was consumed by Lucy's plight. I contacted some of the Chinese women in a local mother's group. They began to support her by taking her shopping and helping to enrol the children in school. She enrolled in a free English class and began to drop into the centre with Peter on a weekly basis. For Lucy, each visit was an opportunity to practise her English.

She had abandoned the long grey overcoat and instead wore jeans and T-shirts. Her long black hair was now bleached blonde, and she wore long dangly earrings.

Now, when she smiled, her eyes twinkled with delight as she told me of her daily discovery of the Western lifestyle that she believed was best for her family.

Today Peter is eighteen months old. As I walk towards the waiting room I hear the voices of Lucy's children playing on the floor with the other children. Lucy is sitting next to a Chinese man and chatting with a Macedonian mother. They are talking about their children's eating habits, and she looks perfectly at ease in her surroundings. As I call her name, Lucy and the man stand up.

'This is my husband,' she says. 'We have come to say goodbye.'

'Are you going back to China?'

Lucy smiles as she explains: 'We have bought a business in Parramatta. We will never go back to China. We are Australian now; we have permanent residency.'

Milk monitor

KATE FIELD

The breastfeeding clinic is often the last resort for mothers. Some of them refer to it as 'milk school'. It's a place where lactation consultants come into contact with a variety of mothers, babies and breasts, and the four of us manage to manoeuvre our way through strategies to suit all involved. People unfairly call us 'nipple nazis'; I like to think that most lactation consultants *support* breastfeeding, rather than enforce it. I am constantly amazed by the stoicism of women in their breastfeeding journeys. Mothers will struggle through weeks of repeated bouts of mastitis, grit their teeth through every feed when their nipples resemble the skinned knees of pre-schoolers, or have voracious babies that demand to be attached permanently to the breast. Then there are the mothers of premature babies who present their invaluable contributions of milk on a daily basis. These women go through weeks, sometimes months, of attaching themselves to a breast pump every few hours. With premature babies surviving at less than 600 grams, breast milk assumes a medicinal role with its anti-infective properties.

On this particular Tuesday, the postnatal ward is busy and three outpatients are booked in. A visit can be as brief as one hour or as long as five hours. Mandy is the first to arrive with her three-week-old son Oscar wedged in a purple sling. She is a first-time mum in her late thirties. The plan today is to wean him off the nipple shield. The much-maligned nipple shield is a useful short-term gadget and often means the difference between weaning or continuing to feed. Mandy had started using the shield a few days after birth with a baby who made no attempt to latch on to her flattish nipples.

Oscar is thriving, well over his birth weight but taking a long time to feed, a common disadvantage with nipple shields. Mandy is nervous about taking off the nipple shield, like driving without a seatbelt.

'I've tried a couple of times, but he gets really frustrated. He shakes his head, like he's saying "No, no, no!" And then he just cracks it,' she explains. 'I don't mind using it, but it's a bit of a nuisance and I left it behind the other day and had to drive all the way back home.'

'It's just a matter of retraining him,' I say. 'Babies are pretty clever. He associates the texture of the shield with getting fed and it's easy for him to grasp.'

Absolute understatement there. Babies aren't pretty clever; in my experience, they're brilliant. A three-day-old baby may already have discovered that its mother's right nipple is easier to latch on to but the left breast produces a faster flow. Babies are the masters of instant gratification. They are the greatest teachers of lactation consultants.

'So,' I continue, 'what we have to do is provide him with something that's just as easy to grasp as the nipple shield.'

Mandy looks doubtful. I produce the demonstration dolly from the cupboard. It looks forlornly at us; someone has put a Collingwood beanie on it and hooked the demo cloth breast around its arm like a shield.

Mandy laughs. The doll and its companion, the appallingly shaped breast, is a fantastic teaching tool but also provides light relief.

'Kate, phone call postnatal desk,' the overhead voice announces.

'Be straight back,' I promise and race off.

'Hello, I need to speak to the lactation person,' says the voice on the end of the phone.

'It's Kate speaking; I'm one of the lactation consultants. And what's your name?'

'Lindy. My baby's six weeks old and I'm feeding him meself,' the young voice continues, 'and when I got up my boob's really red and sore. Me mum told me not to feed the baby 'cos it'll make him chuck.'

I ask a few more questions, reassure her about feeding and speak to Lindy's mother at length. I advise a plan of action and suggest that she ring back in the afternoon if there is no improvement in the symptoms.

Back to Mandy. I'd left her with Oscar just waking. He was now screaming indignantly, unimpressed with the delay.

'Shape your fingers like this, so that they're parallel to where his lips will go. Really over-emphasise the shape for him.'

'Jane, another mum's here,' says the ward clerk, poking her head around the door. 'And the other lady cancelled. She'll come next week.'

A large pram containing an unhappy occupant appears in the doorway, followed by its driver.

'Hi. Janine, is it? I'm Kate. Just take a seat and I'll be with you soon.'

The day stay unit has a different level of workload to other midwifery areas. It often requires intensive care with fractious babies and fragile mothers. We always try to be aware that the feeding issues may be secondary to other problems, such as major adjustment to parenting or postnatal depression. Sometimes the mums just need a shoulder to cry on.

Janine looks pale and tired. She scoops the wailing bundle from the pram and pats it absently.

Mandy's let-down erupts with a vengeance in response to Oscar's nuzzling. The milk sprays all over his face. *Where's that pointy silicone thing?* you can see him wondering.

'Now, as he's opening his mouth nice and wide, compress that shape and bring him on firmly.'

Perfect timing and Oscar sucks furiously for a few minutes before coming off, confused by the new sensation. Mandy latches him again and he slips into the 'third gear' of sucking, deep and rhythmic. He gulps noisily.

She beams. 'That was easy.'

'Some babies get the hang of it really quickly,' I say, crossing my fingers.

I pull a chair over to Janine.

'And how are things going with you, Janine?'

'Not so good. He feeds all the time and he's not putting on any weight. My other boy, he whacked on the weight. I just don't know what to do.' She shakes her head.

'You poor thing,' I say, stroking her arm. 'Is it okay if I have a look at him before he feeds?'

Janine's baby, Brandon, is also three weeks old. Unlike Oscar, though, this one is well below his birth weight. His little brow is compressed into a worried expression, and gangly limbs protrude from his suit. A borderline failure-to-thrive. Despite his leanness, he is bright-eyed with a normal-looking mouth and palate. Nothing obvious to indicate a sucking problem.

Brandon is looking for a feed, so I postpone the history taking to watch him in action. Lactation practice involves observation and patience. He fusses a little to start, then settles into a sucking pattern. There is no 'gear change' into effective sucking with Brandon. His rapid, shallow sucking results in little swallowing and within a few minutes he's closed his eyes, content to obtain whatever trickle of milk he is receiving.

'This is what happens every feed,' says Janine.

With a tired mother of two children under eighteen months, complicated gadgets such as 'supply lines', which supplement the baby through a narrow tube attached near the nipple, aren't a practical option. I run the idea past Janine, but the toddler-friendly aspect of the Lactaid isn't enticing.

'I think the main aims here are to get some more calories into Brandon to give him more energy, and to teach him to latch better to help bump up your supply. If you top him up with some milk after feeds – breastmilk, if you can – he'll start to feed more vigorously.'

I don't mention the 'F' word at this stage. Formula is sometimes a 'necessary evil' if the mother's supply is low. Many mothers will continue to breastfeed for months but give formula as well.

I take the rest of Janine's history, including type of birth, and the feeding pattern in the first week, and start writing a plan for Brandon. In the cot opposite, Oscar is stirring and Mandy wants to try the other side.

'Kate, can you please come to the nursery?' The special care nursery is summoning me. The day stay lounge is at the back of the ward, somewhat isolated.

'Okay, Mandy, same as before. He's looking for that missing nipple shield so shape the breast for him.'

Oscar decides to prove me wrong and launches himself at the breast as though he's never *seen* a nipple shield. He sucks vigorously. His nipple shield addiction is certainly one of the easier ones to discourage.

Janine has occasionally fed her other baby with formula and is happy to feed Brandon small amounts until her supply improves. In view of his shallow breast-feeding attachment, we decide to use a cup rather than a bottle. He takes to the cup readily after a few initial spills, and I feed him while Janine eats her lunch.

'I can't remember the last time I sat down for lunch,' she says.

An impatient voice announces again, 'Kate to nursery, please.' I set Janine up with an electric breast pump and dive into the special care nursery. It's a chaotic jungle of small babies, mothers, midwives, and a doctor's round with a full ensemble of medical students. One of the paediatricians has a captive audience of mothers and students as he practises his recently acquired magic tricks. A coin miraculously appears from a blue silk handkerchief; last week he did card tricks.

'Kylie needs a hand expressing. She's around the back,' says one of the nursery staff.

The mum in question is fifteen, with a two-day-old premature baby. She huddles behind the flimsy curtain clutching a pink teddy and a yellow-topped container.

'They've shown me how to do it, but I can't get any milk out.' She looks about twelve, lost in a foreign place of humidicribs and beeping monitors. A boy, hidden under a black beanie, lounges in a chair, studying the floor. First things first.

'I'm Kate, one of the midwives. Are you happy to try and express some milk for your baby?' I sit on a footstool next to her.

'Yeah, I guess. They said it was good for her,' she adds, twisting the stud in her lip.

'So you had a little girl. What's her name?'

'Taneisha. She's really cute. We bought her this.' She shows me the teddy.

'Because Taneisha's early, your milk is very important to help stop infection,' I explain. 'You might only get little bits to start with, but each drop is full of goodies for her. It's like her first vaccination.'

She looks more interested. I show her where to position her fingers and the direction of pressure. 'I'll be right back,' I say.

It's time to check on outpatient activities. I hope Janine's nipple hasn't been sucked into the tubing by an over-vigorous electric pump!

Janine is intact. Mandy has finished feeding and is booked for a baby massage session. She is keen to leave.

I jot down a few reminder points for her and reassure her that there may be times in the next few days when Oscar will refuse to latch without the shield.

'No, I'm leaving it here,' she says firmly, placing the offending item on the bench.

'It might be handy, just in case,' I warn.

'No, we'll be fine. It really helped coming here today. Good luck,' she says over her shoulder to Janine.

Janine tips a few millilitres of breast milk from the electric pump bottle into a container. 'No wonder he's not putting on weight,' she says ruefully. 'Maybe I should just put him on the bottle.'

'You fed your last one, though,' I point out. 'Let's work out a plan to build up your milk supply, and I'll watch another feed before you go. We'll try and improve his latch. I've just got to check on another mum.'

The young mum in the nursery is squeezing valiantly while leaning over the small jar.

'See, there's nothin' there.'

I readjust her fingers and soon a yellow drop glistens at the tip of her nipple.

'Hey, cool. Look at this, Tim,' she says to her silent boyfriend. She squeezes a few more times, waiting for the drop to fall into the jar. The colostrum clings tenaciously to her nipple, defying gravity.

'Colostrum is very sticky,' I say. I carefully draw the drops off with a syringe.

'You can try a pump when your milk's in. That's a bit easier.'

The other breast is more obliging and produces nearly a millilitre of custard-coloured colostrum. She proudly places the container on top of her baby's isolette.

Janine's baby is asleep, so I turn on a breastfeeding video for her to watch while I squeeze in a late lunch break. It's more like afternoon tea by this stage! When I return, Janine is nodding off in front of the video and smiles apologetically. The luxury of sitting down for longer than fifteen minutes is a forgotten sensation. She is in no hurry to leave, but it's almost 3 pm. After writing her a feeding plan, I send her home with a referral to a speech pathologist and close follow-up from the maternal and child health nurse.

I tidy up the lounge, pack up the breastfeeding gear and return to the office. There's just time to make two follow-up calls to mothers from last week's breastfeeding clinic.

'So, what have you been doing all day?' asks a labour ward midwife as I pull on my coat . . .

A mother's courage

SUE BAKER

It was the phone call I had been expecting. Each day I waited for the news about Simone. Finally, Lisa rang.

'It's happened, Susan. Simone died in the night. Catherine asked me to let you know. The funeral is on Wednesday.'

We spoke for a while, and then I had to take the children to school. Once they were organised and off for the day, there was time for the news to sink in . . .

This all happened six years ago. I had been a maternal and child health nurse for a mere twelve months. Lisa was about to start maternity leave and was handing over to me, so we discussed the routine; all the little things I needed to know about how to run the centre.

Then Lisa pulled out her 'worry file'. All maternal and child health nurses have a worry file, whether it's on paper or in their heads, a file of clients who need extra support and care. Thankfully, this worry file contained only four or five names. As she ran through each of them, I began to relax.

'I can handle this,' I thought. 'Nothing I haven't struck before.'

Then Lisa came to the last family on the list. She sighed and looked at me. 'Oh, this is a hard one for you, Sue. Have you ever wondered if it would be better to just take a pillow and end all the suffering?'

Stunned silence from me. I was quite unnerved, hearing this from Lisa, who isn't prone to exaggeration. This must be really bad.

Catherine's pregnancy had been uneventful. She was only a small woman, but she had already had one child without any complications. She attended all the usual check-ups with her doctor, and nothing had led him to suspect that anything was wrong. Even during the labour all the checks by the midwife indicated everything was progressing normally, and that the mother and baby were coping well.

You see it happen sometimes as a midwife; after the initial elation of the birth, the terrible silence. Then the feverish activity, calling for help, people rushing in, all crowded around the little figure in the cot. Parents not knowing why this was happening. It fills every midwife with dread.

The baby, Simone, did finally breathe, but not for 45 minutes. She was sent to the Children's Hospital in the city, where she was monitored closely. Catherine went with her newborn daughter, while her husband, Tom, stayed home with Beth, their two-year-old.

Simone was a beautiful baby, who looked just like her sister, with masses of wavy black hair, long eyelashes and enormous brown eyes that, you felt sure, saw you and understood. For a few days Catherine didn't know there was anything particularly wrong with Simone. She wasn't having oxygen like the other babies. She didn't need to be in an incubator, either. She had to be given her food through a tube, but so did most of the babies there. She had the usual investigations, but there was no visible clue as to what had prevented her from breathing when she was first born.

Catherine told me later that it wasn't until the paediatrician asked to see her that her world began to fall apart. He told her that Simone had suffered brain damage, and he was unsure what the future held for her. However, they were sent back to their local hospital, where Catherine learned how to tube-feed Simone. A few days later they were able to go home, armed with all the equipment to do the tube-feeding themselves.

Catherine, Tom and Beth settled into the routine of having a new baby in the house. Apart from the fact that Simone's food had to go through a tube, they did all the normal things. They were very busy, but coped well, as Lisa told me during her handover. They had been attending the maternal and child health centre to weigh Simone to ensure that she was being fed enough. Simone never cried if she was hungry, so Catherine had to be very careful that she was feeding her enough.

Lisa went off on her maternity leave, and I took over her position. Catherine and Simone had an appointment to see me later in my first at the centre. Simone was about six weeks old. When Catherine first came in and sat down, my first impression was: 'This is all so normal. Here is a beautiful baby lying in her capsule, next to her mother's chair. Here is a woman who seems just like any other mother.'

Then Catherine began to share her experience with me. Somehow she managed to put on a brave front. In reality, she was up around the clock – tube-feeding and changing Simone every three hours, while also coping with Beth, who was still waking in the night.

Visitors were coming to see the new baby. 'Isn't she beautiful. There can't possibly be anything wrong with her, can there?' one innocently remarked. 'Surely the doctor must be wrong?'

All the while, Catherine could sense that there *was* something wrong. Her precious little girl never cried, never smiled, never acknowledged her mother's touch. She felt torn, because Beth needed her too, but the toddler was spending most of her day watching videos or going out with Dad or Nanna. Catherine didn't have the energy for a two-year-old as well. She was surrounded by people, but she felt alone, trying to cope with the nightmare that her life had become. She was physically and emotionally exhausted.

Okay. This was something I could help with. I organised home care so that Catherine could have some help with feeding Simone and a little of the housework done while she did other things, such as the shopping or keeping appointments for herself. I got Beth an afternoon a week in a creche, so that she would have her own special time with other children, not all these worried adults who kept giving her presents, but didn't play with her like Mummy did. And I arranged to visit Catherine and Simone at home so that she didn't have to struggle with a visit to the health centre in between feeds. It was planned that I would visit twice a week to weigh Simone and monitor her feeding schedule.

I remember exactly where they lived. I could take you there today. It was a little weatherboard house. The garden was immaculate, with annuals planted in a new garden bed out the front. Catherine later told me that the garden kept her sane, and that she often gardened while the home care ladies looked after Simone.

'I only get half an hour, but I feel so much better afterwards,' she said.

A family friend let me into the house. It was obvious that this was a house with children. Toys took pride of place in the lounge. *The Wiggles* was on TV, and a child's scribbly drawing was proudly stuck on the wall. Beth rushed up to see who the visitor was, obviously used to being around adults, and confident that they would have a kind word for her.

Catherine greeted me warmly, and took me into Simone's room. It was all well set up with everything she needed. She had some secondhand things, but it was obvious that her parents had put a lot of time and effort into making her room comfortable. There were three women in blue uniforms fussing around a feeding set, learning how to feed Simone, and family members everywhere. I weighed Simone, and checked that everything was okay. It was impossible to hold a proper conversation in all the chaos. Catherine and I laughed at this, and made an appointment for me to come back at another time. I drove away wondering how she was really coping.

Each week I continued to visit, weighing Simone and making adjustments to her feeding regime as appropriate. We fell into a routine. Some of the visits were more of a chat, nothing much, but I could sense that they were important to Catherine – she wasn't really able to get out much, and we had developed a good rapport. The friends and family had gradually drifted away – nothing was happening, and Catherine really didn't need any help. But it was obvious now that she had time to think. Time to wonder, 'How long will this go on?' and 'Is this what it will always be like?'

By now, Simone should have been smiling back at her mother when she spoke, as other babies did. She should have been able to lift her head, too, but she couldn't. She didn't make any baby noises, either, just a sort of moaning sound.

'I feel as though we're interfering with nature, here,' Catherine said to me one day.

I really didn't know what to say. I couldn't see any alternative.

Catherine took Simone back to see the doctor in the city. She told him she wanted the truth. He gave it to her. She already knew it, but now she heard it said out loud. 'We don't know how long this will go on,' he said, 'but there is no hope. Most of Simone's brain has died, probably long before she was born. Only the part of her brain which controls her most primitive functions survived. She won't ever walk. She won't ever talk.'

On her way home, Catherine decided what she needed to do. *Had* to do, as Simone's mother.

I went to the house a few days after the trip to the city. The house was very quiet. Catherine greeted me at the door before I knocked.

'Hi, Catherine. How was the visit to the paediatrician?' I asked, keen to hear someone else's sense of the situation.

'Not so good, Sue. But it was what we've both been thinking, right?'

'Yes,' I agreed. 'So, what did he say?' We talked about what the doctor had said about Simone's future. Catherine pictured Simone in a wheelchair as a teenager, still in nappies, being fed, just existing, not enjoying the simple things that other children have, such as having friends, going to school, playing sport, having a boyfriend . . . everything that makes life wonderful.

'I don't want that for Simone. And to be honest, Sue, I don't want it for me, or Tom, or Beth.' She paused, then went on with difficulty. 'But I don't know what Simone would want. What do you think?'

Again, I found myself unable to offer a reply.

We went into Simone's room, where she was sleeping peacefully. Catherine picked her up. 'She hasn't fed for six hours. I haven't woken her like I normally do.'

Simone made her usual moaning noise. You were never sure if it meant something.

I watched as Catherine gently changed her nappy and offered her a bottle.

'Where is the tube-feed?' I asked.

Catherine hesitated. 'I'm going to let Simone decide,' she said finally. 'She's got to feed if she wants to live. If not, I will just hold her and love her for as long as I've got her.'

Catherine had been doing this since she had come home from the city. I asked if I could weigh Simone. She had lost 100 grams. Not much. She didn't seem dehydrated. Catherine told me she had been taking about 200 millilitres per day, from feeds that lasted over an hour each time.

It took a while to sink in, that this was the decision she had made. I went away to think about it. At home with my own children that night, slowly I began to understand. Catherine's love and courage just blew me away.

I visited again the next day. Simone was peaceful, as before. Catherine wasn't waking her in the night to feed anymore, but still fed her during the day, every three hours, for as long as she wanted. I weighed her again, and again she had lost weight. Only a little this time, but that was the last time I weighed Simone.

We didn't need to know – and truthfully, I didn't *want* to know.

Catherine went to see her own doctor, and told him of her decision. He understood.

Catherine now had morphine to use if she felt that Simone was suffering, but she hardly ever used it. She wanted it to be Simone's decision when she went. She was comfortable, and surrounded by love. I never, ever saw Catherine cry.

Beth was staying with her nanna, but visiting often. Tom was always there, quietly supportive, making sure that Simone and Catherine had everything they needed. He seemed in awe of his wife's strength. Who knows what he really thought and felt? I hope that someone was supporting him. I continued to visit, every day if I could.

I was moving to another town and a new job in three weeks' time.

'How am I going to leave you, Catherine?' I asked, when I realised that I would be leaving before it was over.

'It's okay. You can go. Just promise me one thing,' she said. 'Come back for the funeral.'

'Of course I will,' I assured her.

A few more visits, and then it was time to say goodbye. I sat in the car outside the house thinking about what to say. I really didn't have any practical advice for Catherine; for a long time she hadn't needed any. But we had formed an understanding. We both knew what was happening. I don't know how many other people did, apart from the doctor.

The home care people were no longer coming. I don't know what they would have thought or done if they had known. Some wouldn't have approved, I'm sure of that. But the love and courage that I saw in that little house will stay with me forever.

'Well, it's goodbye, then.' I held Simone for the last time, and handed her back to Catherine. She gently settled her back into the cot and walked out to the car with me.

'I've got a little gift for you,' she said, and gave me a small package.

We didn't say much, but hugged each other goodbye. I walked straight to the car, not looking back until I was driving down the road. Catherine disappeared back inside. I held her gift in my hand. I didn't feel like I deserved it. I was leaving her now when she needed me the most.

I wore the perfume she'd given me every day. And every day I wondered how they were going, but I never called. I was busy, of course, settling my family into a new house and new schools. And what was there to say? Another nurse was now visiting each day, anyway. I spoke to her and asked how Catherine was coping, and sent her my love, but that was it.

Three weeks later, Simone died.

I hadn't been able to go to the funeral. Or at least I told myself that I couldn't possibly go – it was so far away, and I had to pick the kids up from school anyway. Deep down, I knew I was making excuses. I just couldn't face the flood of emotion I had been holding back for so long. I knew it would all come pouring out if I went to the funeral.

Lisa called me and described what happened. 'Oh, it was hard, Sue. It was so beautiful, but so sad.' She described it in detail for me, and it sounded as though even after she was gone, Catherine kept giving Simone everything that she could. There was Beth's favourite music playing in the chapel. A photo board of the whole family. Balloons. A perfect little white coffin. I wasn't there. I should have been there, but I wasn't.

Several months later, Catherine sent me a letter. And again at Christmas I got a card. Life was returning to a sort of normal for Simone's family, but as Catherine said, it would never be the same. I will always remember Catherine and the incredible love she showed her daughter, by letting her go. Even now, I often think about them, and wonder if they still live in that same little house.

Controlled crying

CHRISTINE CROYDEN

Anne opened the front door, stepped on to the verandah, and took a deep breath of cool morning air. She looked at the newspaper lying at her feet and bent down to pick it up. The creak in her back reminded her that she was alive, although one hour earlier, woken ten times since midnight, she hadn't been sure. A loud squeal came from the kitchen. She ran inside to find her two-year-old standing in his highchair laughing at his sister, who was teasing him with a piece of toast. Frank chomped on his cereal and watched with amusement. He looked at Anne and signalled for the paper. 'Why don't you sit him down? He could fall out,' she said, as she passed it across to him while pushing the squirming toddler back into his seat with her other hand.

'Lighten up. They're just having fun,' Frank said,

raising an eyebrow at the breast poking from her gaping nightie. 'Why don't you buy yourself a new dressing gown? Then if you stay in your bedclothes all day, at least you'll be decent.'

'I would, if I had the chance to go shopping,' she replied.

'What do you do when someone comes to the door?' he said, putting down the paper and reaching for more cereal.

'No one does.'

'Well, why not try to get out of the house and visit somebody . . . or go for a walk in the park?'

She said nothing but sat down opposite him with a heavy thud, buttoned her nightie up to the neck and proceeded to spoon mush into the toddler's mouth. Frank turned to the sports pages. After a few minutes, he raised his head from the paper. 'So, what've you got on for today?'

'Nothing much. I just wish I could stay in bed. I was up all night,' she mumbled as she scraped the last of the baby food from the bowl.

'Really? I didn't hear anything.'

'No, you never do,' she said, scowling. The chance of an argument perked her up for an instant. She opened her mouth to say something further just as Frank rose from the table. 'Okay, I'm off.'

'How bloody convenient,' she muttered.

He leaned over and kissed the top of her head, patted her back, then walked out of the kitchen. A few minutes later she heard the front door slam, followed by a loud squeal from upstairs.

After placing the children in front of *Play School*, Anne dragged herself up the stairs towards the screaming baby.

She stopped and waited on the landing, hoping the sound would cease. It didn't, so she placed one unwilling foot in front of the other until she stood over the crib looking down at the infant, who was writhing and kicking off his bedclothes. When he opened his eyes and saw his mother, a beautific smile lit up his round face. Anne picked him up and placed her cheek on his soft, warm head as he nestled into her shoulder. She stood swaying and felt his heart beating through his jumpsuit and her swollen breasts throbbed. They lay down on the bed together, his eyes fixed on his mother's face as his jaw moved rhythmically between gulping noises. Anne lay back and fell asleep instantly. She woke to find her daughter, Ella, tugging at the doona. 'Muuum! *Play School*'s finished.'

'Shh, Ned's sleeping.' She took her breast from the baby's open mouth and gently placed him back in the cot so that the movement didn't wake him.

'Are the *Bananas* on now?' she whispered to Ella, thinking of taking a shower.

'S'over, too.'

'Okay, let's go and see what James is up to.' She took her daughter's sticky, jam-covered hand and tiptoed out of the room.

Today was the same as yesterday and the day before. On Sunday, Frank had been home and she'd had time to at least read the paper. At 5.30 he'd come in from the garden where he'd spent the whole day, taken the baby from her arms and suggested she go for a walk while he cooked dinner. Anne nodded and went upstairs, pulled on her tracksuit pants and a T-shirt, got a whiff of her nightie, threw it into the wash basket, and left the house for the first time in four days.

As she walked around the park past runners and dogs, she thought about the women she'd nursed all those years ago in the postnatal wards. They'd seemed so hopeless to her then, with their tear-stained faces and exhausted eyes. How could she ever have imagined what it was like? And who could have guessed that ten years and three children later she'd be transformed into one of them? From the self-contained 25-year-old midwife, who had lost patience with women learning to breastfeed, she had become a soft-in-the-middle malcontent, anxious if separated from her children for more than a few hours.

As she walked up the laneway beside their house the smell of smoke from the barbecue wafted over the fence. Frank hadn't cooked a meal since Ned's birth, and the break from their usual diet of pasta with sauce from a jar or rice with leftovers put them both in good spirits for the rest of the evening. After her third glass of red wine they were getting somewhere with a conversation about something other than the children, although she couldn't remember what, when she collapsed into a drunken sleep on the couch.

This morning, Anne was going out with her friend, Sara, for coffee at 11. When she looked at the clock it was ten minutes before the hour and she knew she'd have to call and cancel. The phone rang twice and Sara answered. 'Anne. What's up? Haven't you left?'

'I'm not going to make it this morning. I fell asleep feeding and we're not even dressed yet.'

'Well, mine are in the pram on the verandah and I'm almost out the door,' Sara replied.

'Sorry.'

There was a pause before Sara asked, 'Were you up all night again?'

'Yeah, this baby only sleeps for twenty minutes at a time.'

'I told you to persevere. It works.'

Anne put the phone down and picked up a pencil lying beside it. She began drawing geometric patterns on the blotter. The shapes encroached upon one another. She leaned forward on to her elbows – shading them darker. Controlled crying. She had to harden her heart and do it. Sara was right, it did work for some people – but she hadn't been one of them. After two years of broken sleep with Ella and one-and-a-half with James, perhaps Ned would sleep for the whole night by his first birthday. But he was her last child. Was it necessary to put him through it?

The time she spent breastfeeding him at night was the only quiet time they had together. The others were always at her for something, and if it wasn't them it was Frank. She threw down the pencil and walked into the kitchen. *Who takes care of me?* She opened the fridge and pulled out a plate of cold pasta. She would have been eating a chocolate muffin by now if her coffee morning had eventuated. Anne was enjoying the leftovers when a recognisable smell wafted across from the corner where James was playing with his Duplo. She walked across to the child, swallowing her last mouthful of pasta, and stood above him.

'Is there something in your pants?'

'Nah,' he said, busy trying to secure some red wheels on to the truck he was making.

'Can I have a look?' Anne asked.

He looked up angrily and screamed, 'Nooooo poo!'

She swept him up into her arms and struggled to hold him while he kicked and cried. She pinned him to the floor and changed his nappy, folding it up tightly then pitching it into the laundry where it landed in the bucket with a splosh.

Anne carried him under her arm back to his play corner where he threw himself on to the floor and howled. She looked down with her hands on her hips and was overcome by the desire to smack him, so she left the room and went into the garden. Outdoors, she always felt better. The basket of washing that she'd meant to hang up yesterday sat on a deckchair nearby. She stared at it for a while, then pegged everything neatly on to the line and stood back to admire the job. It was the first task she'd completed to her satisfaction for ages.

She walked around the garden. A few signs of spring poked up among the weeds and a pigeon splashed in the birdbath. The cool air swept over her skin, drawing her out of herself and into the day. She looked up and watched the clouds moving slowly across the sky, then turned towards the door. Inside the house James's crying had stopped, so she tiptoed past the children, who were happily engaged in an imaginary game with Ella's dolls, and went upstairs.

In her room she stretched out on the bed and thought about reading the magazine her sister had bought for her. She lifted her head from the pillow and smelt the dry milk on her bra. She placed her hands on her breasts to feel them – at least they weren't leaking. Her other bras were on the line, so this dirty one would just have to do.

Anne caught a glimpse of herself in the mirror and a puffy, dishevelled woman in a flannelette nightie looked back. The sight brought hot tears to her eyes. She lay back and let them flow.

That evening, after the dinner circus, she flopped into her favourite chair with the baby on her lap for the before bed feeding session. Frank poured her another glass of wine. She took a few large gulps. He watched, holding the bottle in mid-air, then said: 'Sip it. You'll be asleep by eight at this rate.'

'Oh, give me a break,' she replied. After a more restrained swallow, she added: 'This isn't bad.'

'Exactly. That's why you sip it.'

He walked across the room towards the couch and placed the bottle on the table. He picked up the remote control. 'You know, I never heard my mother complain once,' he said, his eyes fixed on the TV screen. They sat watching in silence until Anne's eyes began to close. She pulled herself up and laid the sleeping baby on the couch beside her.

'What do you think about trying control crying tonight?' she said.

'Why? It doesn't work.' After a moment, he added: 'We can do it if you like, but I can't get up. I have an early start tomorrow.'

'Well, you'll have to, otherwise it won't work. He smells the milk on me and it makes him scream more.'

'On the weekend.'

'No. Tonight.'

'Okay,' he conceded, glancing tenderly at the sleeping

baby beside her on the couch. 'Do you want me to take him upstairs?'

'Yes. I think I'll have a bath,' she said, pulling herself out of the chair.

That night she lay in bed waiting for the crying to begin. Frank snored softly beside her. Then it came, the first whimpering, which gradually wound up to a full-force cry. She lay still holding her breath and looked at the clock, nudging Frank.

'It's two o'clock and he's awake.'

'Yeah, so we leave him to scream it out for twenty minutes,' he replied.

Her throat tightened and her skin prickled. The crying became more distressed. After ten minutes the baby was losing steam but still whimpering. Every so often the noise stopped. She tried to loosen her body by rolling from side to side and opening and closing her mouth to release her jaw. The crying ceased.

Anne got up and tiptoed to the entrance of the baby's room next-door. She stood and listened for the sound of breathing and could just discern it above the pounding of her own heart. She climbed into bed and held on to Frank's bare back and waited. Fifteen minutes later it began again, rapidly revving into full distress. She felt milk trickling into her armpits and a physical ache somewhere in her gut. She wanted to pick him up. Frank turned towards her and held her wrist.

'Stay here, he's almost out of puff. Can't you hear it? He needs to sleep as much as we do.'

'I can't stand this,' she whispered.

'Just give him five more minutes.'

The baby stopped again. Quiet. The sound of the clock ticking, five minutes passed, no more noise. She pulled the pillow over her head and fell into a deep sleep.

The crying entered her consciousness before her memory told her to stay put. She jumped out of bed, then hesitated, realising she had meant to leave him again, and got back under the covers. Frank was really snoring; this bout of crying wouldn't wake him. It escalated into a choking raw sob. She needed to hold him and touch his wet, soft face. In her nightmares she'd often hear her children cry but she was never able to reach them.

No child of mine shall be left to cry alone in the dark. Anne sat up and kicked off the doona.

Names have been changed in this story.

A dirty secret

SUSAN TIMPANI

I fixed my attention on Sister Gertrude's hands as she mimicked delivering a baby. With one hand she supported the mother's perineal muscle, while easing the baby's head out with the other. Sister then folded her arms across her generous bosom. The tension in her voice was apparent.

'A perineal tear is sometimes unavoidable.' We felt her eyes roll across our group of trainee midwives. 'However, a *third* degree tear is a mortal sin!' She grasped her large silver cross dangling between her breasts. 'Failing to detect it at delivery is worse. It is unforgivable!'

Many years later, my best friend and colleague, Fiona, could bear testimony to this. We worked together in the labour ward until she left on maternity leave.

One morning when I came on duty, I read Fiona's name on the in-patient board. When I entered her room she was grasping her knees to her chest. Harrowing moans escaped her clenched jaw as she bore down. I tiptoed closer and laid my hand on her shoulder. 'It looks like it won't be long.'

I greeted Ken, Fiona's husband.

'We've been here all night.' Ken's bulky hands smoothed Fiona's forehead with the cool face washer. 'I just wish it was over.'

Doctor Graham stood at the foot of the bed, clad in a green surgical gown and disposable gloves. Therese, the night midwife, placed a pair of large metal forceps on to the delivery tray. Fiona opened her eyes and relaxed her legs. 'I've been pushing for ages, Sue.' Her voice was faint. 'But my baby just won't turn.'

The doctor picked up a syringe with a long needle attached. He looked up. 'Since you chose not to have an epidural, I'll have to use this to numb the nerve in the pelvic floor.'

Ken and I offered support for Fiona over the next few contractions. 'Come on, Fi. Breathe in the gas,' I coaxed. The nitrous oxide wafted around the head of the bed as she inhaled erratically. '*You* need it, not *us*!' Suddenly Fiona gave an ear-piercing screech.

'I've just turned baby's head manually and I'm now using the forceps,' the doctor said.

Fiona was finally rewarded as he lifted the wet and slippery baby boy on to her tummy.

'You'll need a few stitches,' Doctor Graham mumbled after a brief examination.

A few stiches.

Therese, the midwife looking after Fiona, looked down at the tear and then up at me. Her wide eyes told me the perineum was a shocking mess.

A few months later, Fiona and I sat at her kitchen table sipping rich percolated coffee. The baby slept. I leaned back, relishing the hush that follows a settled baby. I picked up the thread of our conversation.

'Why won't you come shopping when Caleb wakes up?' I persisted.

Our two cups clinked together as Fiona snatched them up. She yanked the tap lever and water splashed over the sink and down her shirt.

'I can hardly even go out for a walk, Sue.' She grabbed the green tea towel, drying herself vigorously. 'I've been shopping once since Caleb was born and it was the worst thing that's ever happened to me.'

She came back to the table and, avoiding my eyes, fixed hers on the sugar bowl. Fiddling with its lid, she told me her story.

'It was the first time I had gone food shopping since Caleb was born. The trolley was as full as it could get, around his capsule. All of a sudden I had to go to the loo, and I needed to get there straight away.' Fiona looked up at me. 'And it wasn't just for a wee.'

She looked out the window. 'I held my breath trying to hold on, praying that the feeling would pass, but it just got worse. I was panicking and trying to think at the same time. The toilet was down the other end of the mall. Caleb's capsule was too heavy and I knew I wouldn't make it if I tried to pick it up. I thought of snatching

Caleb out of his capsule and making a dash through an open checkout.'

Fiona turned back to me. 'But what was I supposed to do with him when I got there? Put him on the floor?'

'That's such a horrible experience!' I passed my friend the tissue box.

Wiping her nose and eyes, Fiona hid behind the tissue. 'Before I knew it, it was too late,' she said. 'Loose faeces were leaking out of me. I pushed the trolley straight to the checkout to pay and get out of there. The woman was fussing over Caleb and when she handed me the change she said: "You better get him home and change his nappy, love."'

I was furious at what Fiona was going through and my mind went back to Caleb's birth. 'It's obvious what's happened,' I told her.

Fiona looked blank.

'Those *few* stitches you had at delivery weren't enough,' I said. 'I reckon you must have torn right up to the back passage and that doctor didn't notice.'

'*A third-degree tear*?' She stared at me.

I nodded. 'A scan will show it up for sure, but it makes sense.'

We both looked out the window for a moment, then I braved another question. 'What about Ken? Does this affect, you know, the two of you?'

We laughed together, glad to dispel some of the seriousness in the air.

'*Everything's* been affected. First of all, I'm not the same stunning, untainted woman that he married.' She smiled at her weak attempt at humour. 'Or so it feels. It's like I've been violated, that a whole part of me isn't private or sacred anymore. I'm paranoid that I'm not clean, or I might have an accident. This makes it all such an effort. When we do give it a go, it hurts like mad.' She sighed. 'Dyspareunia, they call it. So terribly clinical. If only they knew what it really means for a couple.'

She stood up. 'Why don't we sit outside in the sun?' It was a distraction from such an intimate and painful topic. 'You can sit on the rocker.' Fiona pointed to the wicker rocking chair on the porch, settling herself on a well-padded lounge chair.

'Ken and I bought the rocking chair from a second-hand shop last year. When I was pregnant, I dreamt of the day that I would breastfeed him to sleep. Now it feels like I'm rolling on a bed of marbles.'

Caleb's cries from the back room interrupted our conversation.

'I can only breastfeed him lying down,' Fiona told me.

There were just so many consequences of a third-degree tear. I hugged her goodbye, promising to give her a call.

A week later I phoned.

'You were right,' she told me. 'The opening of the bowel is so wrecked that there's only about a third of the original muscle left. They sent me to this colorectal surgeon who told me flat out that he wouldn't even think about repairing it if I'm going to have more children.'

I couldn't believe it. Both she and Ken had planned on having a large family, at least four children.

'I can't not have any more kids,' she said, her voice cracking. 'I'm just going to have to go on living like this.'

'Can't you just avoid deliveries by having Caesareans?' I said, trying hard to find other options for her.

'He said the weight of the pregnancy and the action of the hormones alone could be enough to undo the repair. If that happens, there will no muscle left at all to attempt more surgery.' I wondered if she ought to try a second opinion, but I knew she had made up her mind.

Fiona attempted to work casual shifts when Caleb was around nine months old. During one lunchbreak at work she told me that she couldn't continue to nurse in a hospital.

'We're on our feet for hours, with stops and starts as you move around the ward. This is the perfect condition for constant motility of the bowel – it just keeps pushing faeces along. On a bad day I can go to the toilet up to ten times. Sometimes there's only the two of us on a shift and it's just not safe to leave that person while I run off to the loo. Then there's patient care. I set up the delivery trolley, the resuscitation trolley and the baby's just about to deliver and suddenly I have to tell everyone to hang on because I can't hang on!'

She laughed, but I knew it was a very sad day for her.

Fiona and I lost touch for a while, but I met her again at a hospital reunion for staff and their families. When I saw her with four children in tow I knew that the intervening years must have had their challenges. After a few glasses of white wine, and with the children seated in front of a *Harry Potter* video, we shared where life had taken us.

'We had all our children within five years!' Fiona told me.

'You've got to be kidding!'

'We figured the sooner the better, and then get on with fixing up my plumbing. I had normal deliveries and not a Caesarean because I couldn't bear the thought of another wound on my body. Both deliveries were very quick and we didn't have time to talk about an episiotomy. I'm really glad, because all I sustained were mild tears. The perineal muscle has actually healed very well.' She took a large sip of her wine, and paused.

'I wish I could say the same for the other. The surgeon did what he could but it's far from perfect. My children complain that I can't go shopping without making at least two trips to the loo. I've had to explain that it's a health problem and that's just the way it is. They've been pretty good since then. From experience I know which of the smaller shopping centres don't have toilets, and so I avoid them.'

I asked her about work.

'Yes, I'm working again now, in an obstetrician's private rooms. On the odd occasion I work a hospital shift to keep up my acute skills. Then I dose myself up with anti-diarrhoeal medication, paying the price the next day when everything gushes back to normal! I pretty well know all the triggers and that's helped me have a fair bit of . . . you know . . . control.'

We laughed at the pun, and placed our empty glasses on the table.

'So, all's well that ends well?' I challenged her. It was great to hear of her courage, but I wasn't convinced that she had completely accepted the impact of that tear.

'Almost. I take one tablet that a doctor suggested every day and that's made a huge difference.' She looked over at the children before looking frankly at me again. 'Sure, there are times when it's as bad as it was in the beginning. Last year, our family stayed in a caravan park. The toilet and shower block was totally inadequate for the number of people staying there. Long queues, ice-cold water and less than perfect hygiene made it an absolute nightmare. Over the years, doctors have offered me various suggestions. A colostomy was one proposal. He said to me: "At least you'll have some say in the where and when of your toilet stops."'

'You're kidding!' I said again, by now quite light-headed. 'What did you say?'

Fiona stared at me as if I was nuts. '*You're kidding*, that's what I told him. At another consult with him, he talked about a new treatment where they insert a pacemaker into the bowel to send it messages at a programmed rate or something. "Have you put one in before?" I asked him. "One patient, and it didn't help," he admitted. I said: "Forget it!"'

She paused. 'Sue, do you remember how Sister Gertrude used to rave on about third-degree tears?'

'How could I forget?'

'About how they can be prevented, or detected and reported?'

I nodded.

'She was right,' Fiona continued. 'If a tear isn't dealt with properly, it's far worse for mothers than for the staff. It's the mothers who have to live with the dirty secret.'

Baby Royal

ROBIN BARKER

I'm on my way to visit Boris, Leanne and baby Royal.

Royal is named after the maternity hospital where he was born because Boris and Leanne had such a positive birth experience there. Three of us – Bill the mental health nurse, Cathy, the Family and Child Services officer (FACS) and Robin, the patron saint of mothers – are involved in their care. As far as I'm concerned it wouldn't matter if twenty people were involved in their care, it wouldn't be enough.

Boris Farmer is around 40 and has schizophrenia. Originally from Darwin, he turned up at the Community Mental Health Centre about seven years ago, barefoot and raving during a psychotic episode, and he's been on Bill's books ever since. According to Boris, earlier in his life he alternated between being a naturopath and a chiropractor. He loves prescribing herbal treatments and getting his hands on people to 'crack' their bones. Bill says that Boris is intelligent, charming, even charismatic, when he's well, but when he goes off his treatment he can be frightening, occasionally violent. He took to Bill with a kitchen knife once. He is also a big dope smoker, which doesn't help.

Leanne Driver is intellectually challenged, or whatever the politically correct term is. That is, she has a low IQ – or as Bill once commented, much to Cathy's dismay, 'Leanne is two sandwiches short of a picnic.' She is apparently completely under Boris's spell. Before she met him she'd had two other babies, both removed from her care. She and Boris have been together for a couple of years, mostly hanging out in a cave in the local park until FACS organised a nice Department of Housing flat for them right on the beachfront – excellent views.

I find Boris and Leanne's flat in a small block tucked in between a couple of houses. A fresh spring breeze full of the smell of the ocean and the rogue freesias sprouting up on the nature strip blows into my face. I wouldn't mind living here myself. Boris opens the door with a flourish.

'Robin!' he says. 'Please come in.'

He's tall, sinewy and powerful – you wouldn't want to get on the wrong side of him – with straw hair sticking out at all angles, a beak of a nose red from the sun, and big bone-cracking hands. He's wearing old-style leather sandals and a grubby sarong, and holding a branch aloft. The effect is overwhelmingly biblical – Moses or John the Baptist.

I follow him down a short hallway past a kitchen

where there's something bubbling on the stove in a huge pot. He takes a quick detour, rips some leaves off the branch, pops them into the pot and throws the branch on to a pile of foliage on the floor.

'Nutrients,' he says. 'You can live on what you find growing wild. And lantana juice is a great liver cleanser. Tea or coffee?'

His smile is engaging. I get a sense of the charisma factor. 'No, no thanks, Boris. I just wanted to drop in, congratulate you on the arrival of . . . ' – I stumble a little – '. . . Royal, and say hello to Leanne.'

The baby Royal lies on a blanket, arms and legs waving, and Leanne is kneeling over him crooning. I squat down beside them. 'What a gorgeous baby.' It comes out as a phoney gush. Sometimes I embarrass myself.

Leanne has black curls, very pale skin and big yellow teeth. Her smile is pleasant, if a little loose and wet.

'He's a real good baby,' she says. 'Never cries.' She plops out both breasts. 'My nipples are sore.'

Boris stands over us, legs apart, arms folded. 'I've told her to put mashed nasturtium leaves on them, Rob, and they've improved out of sight.'

Rob? Mashed nasturtium leaves? Well, why not.

'Can I pick Royal up?'

The baby feels good, like he's getting plenty of milk. His skin is pink, eyes clear. He clutches my finger. He's got Boris's narrow face and Leanne's black hair.

'Is he doing plenty of poo?'

Boris is on the floor now looming in between Leanne and me. He takes up a lot of personal space, which I find vaguely intimidating. 'The bowels are good, Rob. I do a bit of tummy massage and a little bit of hip manipulation.'

I hand Royal back to his mother. She squashes him into her breasts. 'Go gently on the chiropractic, Boris,' I say as tactfully as I can. 'He's only a baby. Breastfed babies poo okay without any help.'

Boris flaps his hands in front of my face. 'These, Rob, are the hands of a healer with a velvet touch. You oughta let me give you the once-over. I sense the stress in you.'

We stumble along for the first eight weeks. Cathy is cautiously optimistic, I'm constantly worried about them, and Bill is happy that Boris is still fronting up regularly for his injections. They make it to the centre most weeks. When they don't turn up, I go to the flat. I have to constantly persuade Boris that his proposed treatments – lantana juice for Royal's 'allergic' rash, Weetbix in soy to help him sleep at night, oil of cloves for teething, and mashed cabbage for his cradle cap – aren't appropriate for babies. Boris assures me that the cradle cap is a sign of the toxins coming out. Leanne gives up on the breastfeeding in about week six and I spend a morning with them showing them the intricacies of formula feeding. Despite my concerns, Royal is gaining weight and developing well – bright and alert, cooing, good muscle tone. He's a dear little baby, patient and undemanding, and by now I'm even used to his name.

Christmas approaches. It's a time of the year when there is a risk of everything going pear-shaped because of the public holidays and the tradition in community health of giving leave to any staff who want it. Bill, Cathy and I have a meeting. Bill and I are off for three weeks and Cathy is off for six weeks, which means we've got two weeks not covered. Surely Boris and Leanne can manage for two weeks? I mean, how long is this close supervision going to go on for? The rest of their lives?

A few weeks later, when Boris and Leanne don't turn up for an appointment, I drop in to the flat. No one is home. It's a blazing, eye-squinting December day with a cloudless sky and a sun fierce enough to take off two layers of skin. I wander down the side of the path to the back of the flats. On a patch of grass between two clotheslines lie Boris and Leanne on sheets of silver foil. Glistening oil gathers in thick globules all over their bodies; eyeshades cover their eyes. Boris has leathery skin, but Leanne's whiteness has turned bright pink which continues to deepen as I watch. She is topless, her blue-veined breasts flattened out like plates.

'Hi, you two. How are you going?'

Boris raises the eyeshade, leaps to his feet and smacks his hip as if reaching for a gun. His gaze is hard and flat. For a moment I'm not sure if he sees me. Leanne doesn't move.

He blinks and focuses. 'Rob, Rob, Rob.' He runs his hands down his torso smoothing out the blobs of oil. 'You gave me a fright.' Now his eyes won't meet mine. I feel a tiny thrill of alarm.

'Where's Royal?'

'Inside, Rob. Having his nap. We're taking the opportunity to do a bit of detoxing.'

'Leanne,' I raise my voice. 'Don't you think you've had enough sun? You'll get sick if you stay out here in this.'

Leanne raises the eyeshade and stares at me with blank, watery eyes.

I nearly lose it. 'Did you both forget your appointment yesterday? You know it's important to keep the appointments, because if you want to keep Royal that's part of the deal.'

I step back just in time to escape Boris's big oily hand clapping my shoulder.

'Rob, apologies. We had to go to the doctor. Royal had a little pain in his tummy. Dr Ho gave us some herbal medicine, sorted him right out. I was gunna ring you.'

We troop inside. The flat seems to be getting more and more chaotic. The living room is clogged with newspapers and boxes, clothes are draped over chairs, and there's a strange smell of decomposing vegetation.

Royal wakes up when we go into his room where, surprisingly, order seems to prevail. There's an array of soft toys lined up against a wall, and a tricycle and a pick-up truck by the cot. I take Royal out into the light and examine him carefully. He feels muscular and warm, his skin is firm and rosy, his eyes glisten, he smiles like there is someone at home. I sit Boris and Leanne down and step by step check on the feeding, the poo, the sleeping. I keep telling myself that while Boris might have a mental health problem and is eccentric, he's not stupid. And plenty of people live in chaotic homes, especially when a baby comes into their lives. Before I leave I ask to see the herbal medicine. It's Phenergan, a sedative.

I try for a tone of confiding Aussie blokiness. 'Now, Boris, mate, this isn't herbal. It's a sedative. Very dangerous for babies. I think if you don't mind I'll pour it down the sink.'

Boris's jaw tightens, his eyes go beady. 'It helps his tummy. We only give him a few drops.'

He glares at me. I drop the blokiness and take a firm stand. 'I don't think Cathy will be too happy when I tell her about this.'

Boris's face is like concrete. Leanne tilts her head to one side and looks defiant. Wrong approach. I try flattery. 'Look, you two, you're taking such good care of Royal it would be a shame if there was an accident with the sedative. Let's chuck it out, and when you come to see me tomorrow so that I can weigh Royal I'll give you something else that will work just as well but isn't dangerous. Okay?' I say, taking the Phenergan to the sink. 'Okay?'

Boris shrugs, takes the lid off the pot on the stove and pushes at the contents with a potato masher. 'You're the boss, Rob. Coffee?'

I just want to get out, but it's crucial to keep the communication open. I want to make sure they get to the centre in the morning. 'Thanks, Boris. That would be lovely.'

Leanne and I make faces at Royal while Boris organises the coffee. 'Milk, Rob?'

'Yes, indeed.'

I watch as Boris prises open a big tin of formula, scoops out a heaped spoon of powder, stirs it into the coffee and pushes it towards me.

'Thanks, Boris,' I say.

I check with Bill that Boris is still fronting for his injections. He is, and he and Leanne keep their appointments with me right up until the week I go on leave at Christmas.

The week I go back to work is hot and steamy. The gentle spring breezes have turned into blustering winds heavy with salt and the occasional blast of sewage. There's a constant stream of mothers and babies, and the phone never stops ringing. The days are long and the notion of a lunch hour is a joke. Thankfully, Karen, Cathy's replacement, offers to drop in on Boris and Leanne.

When she calls me, her voice is tense. 'Robin, I'm bringing Royal down to the centre right now. I hope that's okay.'

'Of course it is. Everyone will just have to wait.'

Karen, carrying a baby capsule with Boris and Leanne in tow, pushes her way through a sea of resigned-faced mothers and bug-eyed babies. We assemble in my office. Karen passes me an empty bottle. 'I think you need to examine Royal.' Her eyes are a mixture of shock and anger.

Pressure builds up around my ribs. I take the phone off the hook and reach down for Royal.

Oh, Royal, what have they done to you? Gaunt and grey, he looks like an old man, his mouth locked into a tight grimace. His eyes are enormous and even though they are listless and, it seems to me, full of despair, a flicker of life responds when I whisper to him. I lift him on to the examination table and undress him. I can feel all his bones shifting beneath the skin, stretched tight in some places, hanging limply in others. A line of scabs runs down his spine. When I put him on the scales he puts his hand to his mouth and sucks at his fingernails, long and curving, uncut for weeks.

'He's just on 3 kilos,' I say. 'Way underweight for a four-month-old baby.' I look at the empty bottle. Phenergan.

Leanne is sitting down, head bowed, plucking at her shirt, refusing to look at anyone. Boris takes a lunge towards me. Karen, a big girl in jeans and clunky big-soled shoes, steps in between us and Boris grabs the desk instead.

'What do you recommend, Robin?' Karen's voice is unnaturally loud.

'Immediate admission to the Children's Hospital. I'll call them so they know you're coming. Obviously, it's a matter for Child Protection. I can't imagine . . ' my voice tails off.

I can't imagine anyone in their right senses allowing these two to ever have permanent care of a baby again. I feel outraged, distressed, self-righteous, defensive and, worst of all almost paralysed by a great galloping siege of guilt. We didn't do enough. Christmas we dropped the ball, no one visited them for four weeks which was long enough for a catastrophe. Thank God Karen went when she did; there is, after all, a worse scenario.

Karen has Royal back in the capsule.

'Well, we're coming too,' I hear Boris say. 'I don't trust doctors. They use too many drugs.'

'Of course,' Karen says smoothly. 'Of course, you must come. You are, after all, Royal's parents.'

Finding her way

JAN ROUGHLEY

Kelly had been home from hospital for three days following the birth of her baby Joshua when I first met her. Her mother, June, was very warm and inviting when I arrived at the house and very proud to show me Joshua, her newborn grandson.

They all lived with Rose, Kelly's grandmother. The house was like many others in the area – red brick, wire fence and driveway down the side, a few hardy plants around the front door. Once inside there was an opportunity for an individual stamp to be put on their home. I was led into a neat and orderly living area with just enough furniture to fill the small space. A few trinkets and photos of Kelly were displayed above the gas heater. Rose was welcoming – 'you can sit in the comfy chair' – but was otherwise happy to stay in the background. Kelly had become a mother at just sixteen.

June doted on the precious bundle that lay restfully in her daughter's arms. Kelly herself answered my questions politely, but I sensed the wariness in her that I've become accustomed to in working with adolescent mothers. Often, they're hesitant to let new people into their lives, cautious about unfair, judgmental attitudes. I learned that Joshua's father, Dave, visited regularly and wanted to be part of his son's upbringing. June and Rose were quiet but attentive throughout our conversation, keeping their eyes on Kelly and her new baby. June was keen to point out that everything would be okay.

'She's a good mum and we are always around to help her out,' she said.

Joshua stirred and tentatively opened his eyes. With no hesitation, Kelly confidently breastfed him. He drank contentedly as she smiled and became more relaxed as the discussion shifted to Joshua. I did a preliminary examination and arranged for Kelly to bring Joshua for his two-week assessment at the maternal and child health centre.

It seemed to me to be a supportive home environment for Kelly, one where she could get some rest and care for Joshua without the pressures that some adolescent parents face. In the new realm between adolescence, adulthood and parenting, many young people succumb to despair when faced with the demands of caring for a child. They feel keenly the loss of having somebody to care for them. Sometimes, homelessness compounds all their other problems. Kelly was in a comparatively good situation.

Kelly brought Joshua to the maternal and child health centre regularly, and over time her story unfolded.

'Mum's intellectually disabled, but she's wonderful helping me with Joshua. She can get the bus to the shops, do the cooking and cleaning, but can't manage the bills. Once the phone got disconnected because Mum left the phone bill in Gran's room, but she ignores bills. The phone company wouldn't let me reconnect without speaking to Gran, because it's in her name.'

June and Rose relied on Kelly's common sense in managing the family budget. Rose had always helped June with Kelly's upbringing, but her legacy of many years of narcotic drug use and heavy smoking meant she now relied on Kelly to attend to the family's needs.

Kelly loved talking about Joshua's progress and eagerly collected any written information about immunisation, development, behaviour and play. She made sure she was always well informed so that she could make the best choices for her son and herself. She seemed so organised for a sixteen-year-old, bringing a folder each visit to file away new brochures enthusiastically, and was always interested in listening to the opinions of others. She was wise and honest enough to say, 'I don't know.' And when it came to Joshua's wellbeing, she was determined to learn.

I was rarely offered an insight into Kelly's world. I feared that she'd been made to shoulder so much responsibility that her family's needs might override her own. I always asked her about this and she was very honest in her responses, but didn't seem to see this as important. We spent our time discussing Joshua's growth and development as he giggled, babbled, and started crawling and sitting like any other healthy baby during those first eight months of life. His distinct personality began to emerge, and we discussed behaviour and what to expect from a child who was ready to explore without any fears.

'Is it alright to breastfeed when Joshua cries in the afternoon? Mum keeps telling me to try formula because that was what I was given. She can't wait to feed him.'

Food was always a hot topic. June and Rose insisted on a diet that Kelly had been offered in her first year, which included custard every day and bottles of juice. This caused some conflict, but June and Rose treated Kelly's final decisions with respect.

Kelly had remained close to a small group of friends from school, and they appeared to provide some balance to her readily adopted adult responsibilities. Sometimes, listening to her, it was hard to imagine how she had developed so much maturity in her short life. She found her own way, by thinking with clarity and honesty, and had the security of a loving family.

Joshua was now her main focus, and it soon became apparent that he needed a lot of time and attention. As with most six-month-olds, he spent longer periods awake and started rolling around the room.

Kelly was wanting to move, too. 'I'm going to live with Dave, but I'll keep helping Mum and Gran with their bills and making sure they're alright,' she told me. 'I'll probably see them most days, anyway, because I'll only be around the corner and Mum will want to see Joshua.'

You would think that, to an adolescent, this would seem like a millstone around their neck; to Kelly, shouldering the responsibility for her mother and grandmother seemed as natural as breathing.

She and Dave moved into a unit together, and in this changed family environment another layer of Kelly's wise and resilient self unfolded, as she strove to maintain harmony among everyone's different needs. Dave's job was based locally, but he spent several nights away each week, travelling around Victoria. When he was home, he enjoyed catching up with his mates, which meant social drinking and smoking sometimes at their house. Kelly preferred not to be a part of this. She worked part-time from home, gluing production-line components together. As informed as ever, she was concerned that Joshua was being exposed to cigarette smoke and glue fumes due to her home-based work. She made sure he slept with his door closed and window open prior to the evening's activities, and kept the house well ventilated with windows open in the evening and morning before Joshua got out of bed.

I never had any concerns for Joshua. He always had lots of cuddles, and was always with Kelly or June, being shown the world around him.

Kelly, independent and determined, continued to keep her life to herself. She had left school in Year 9 and I asked her if she thought about further education. 'I passed Year 9 because my marks had been good enough to get a pass and I'm doing Year 10 by correspondence. Mum's been helping by taking Joshua some afternoons.'

She didn't mention it again, but some months afterwards, I discovered she had received 'A's for the first two subjects. Even though it was unheralded, it was a wonderful acknowledgment of the quiet strength of character of a truly amazing young woman. Kelly's maturity and resilience, and her acceptance of the complexities of life, ensured that those she loved were comfortable and happy.

It's a privilege to share with people the transition to parenthood and the expansion of the family. It's a time of growth, many changes and a lot of stress. An experience where we can be guides for part of one of life's most challenging, yet rewarding, journeys. Many years later, I still sometimes wonder where Kelly's journey has taken her.

Blue balloons on the farm gate

LYN HOFFMAN

You can always tell if you're getting close to the right house out in the country, even if you can't quite understand the 'mud map': *Go past the round hay bales on the left side of the road, and next turn right, past the big clump of bullrushes. . .* The sure give-aways are the rows of nappies on the clothesline flapping in the breeze, or the blue balloons on the farm gate. In town, it's a more subtle sign: the 'It's a girl' poster in the window, or a pink bow on the letterbox . . .

5 June, 0800 hours

Pick up two new referrals that went home yesterday evening from the postnatal ward, check that the Central

Health Interpreter Service was booked for the 1100 hours visit, make a few phone calls, and sort out the client rounds for the day. Turn over the sign in the ward to say: 'Domiciliary Midwife is Out on the Road', and off I go for the day.

0845 hours, 32,300 kilometres

Three degrees Celsius. Brrrr! Frosty night last night, fill up the cordial bottle with water from the tap to get the ice off the car, hope the fog clears soon . . .

0855 hours, 32,301 kilometres

First visit to Jenny and Tom, preschooler Sarah and newborn Benjamin, Day 4. Went home Day 2 postnatal, confident mother, breastfed the first child for ten months. Main concern is Benjamin was looking quite yellow when I did the neonatal screening test yesterday, so I put him first on my list today.

'How has he fed overnight?'

'Not too well – he's very sleepy.'

'He definitely looks more jaundiced today – sorry, but I'll have to bleed him again today for a serum bilirubin test. He may need to be readmitted to hospital.'

I again discuss the causes and possible outcomes of neonatal jaundice.

Sarah had been at kinder yesterday, so was very interested in my visit – 'What's in that box? Can Dolly have her blood pressure checked? Can I get on the weigher, too?'

Jenny said, 'Sshhh, Sarah, not so many questions. Please just sit and watch.'

Things are going well until I do the blood test. Benjamin starts crying, which frightens Sarah, so she cries, too. The wails increase, and it's all too much for Jenny who is a bit tired and feeling down. I notice a few tears rolling down her cheeks, as she holds Benjamin for me. Blood test finished, Tom to the rescue – cuppa for Jenny, cuddle for Benjamin, breakfast for Sarah. Thanks, Tom!

Will phone later with the results . . .

0945 hours, 32,302 kilometres

I drop off Benjamin's blood to pathology for the test – marked 'urgent'. Phone call to next client: 'Please take some painkillers – I'll be there soon to take the clips out.'

1000 hours, 32,304 kilometres

'Hi, come in. This is Auntie Violet, my mum Mary, my sister Rochelle, and the kids are all out the back playing.'

I'm at Shannon's unit. She is Day 5, emergency Caesarean section, third baby, and of Aboriginal descent. The families of our local Koori population are usually well supported by a close family network and the local indigenous health system. Baby Crystal gaining weight/feeding well/no concerns. Grandma is having a nurse during my visit.

'Shannon's hair looked just like that when she was a baby,' she says wistfully as she strokes the soft black fluffy locks.

We go into the bedroom and check the wound. Clips all due to be taken out today. Shannon is a bit nervous;

the other two had been normal births. The wound is tender, with signs of infection at the right side. Slowly and gently I take out the staples – fourteen in all. We count as we go. I collect a wound swab to send to pathology and discuss wound care.

Will be in touch when the results come through and get the doctor to order some antibiotics . . .

1100 hours, 32,306 kilometres

I make it just in time to meet the interpreter. But where is the female interpreter I had requested for my Muslim client? Sorry, she was unavailable. They had sent me a man! Due to religious beliefs, Muslim women show a marked preference for female healthcare providers.

Nevertheless, as we kick off our shoes, we are met at the door by husband Hamid and ushered into the lounge room. I apologise for the lack of a female interpreter, but Hamid seems okay with the situation. We sit on mattresses on the floor and admire the pictures on the wall complete with Arabic inscriptions. Hamid's wife Esra appears in her flowing mauve robes and head cloth, followed closely by daughters Fatima and Aeman, and son Ali.

'You want hot drink or Pepsi?' she asks. I reply that Pepsi will be fine.

Via the interpreter, Hamid tells us that the family are originally from Iraq. He had been in the Woomera Detention Centre and his wife and children had been sent to Nauru. He is grateful to now be living in Shepparton, and the local Ethnic Council has been helpful in settling them into the community. As we speak, three little pairs of dark eyes sit in a row in front of me and speak not a word. Esra appears with the can of Pepsi and a glass on the mandatory 'silver' platter and we have a drink as Hamid passes around the glass bowl filled with caramel toffees.

We briefly chat about the events surrounding baby Mohammed's birth and then, as if on cue, he wakes up for a feed. Not wanting to breastfeed in front of a strange male, Esra excuses herself and retreats to the bedroom, leaving me in the lounge with Hamid and the interpreter. I then also excuse myself and go into the bedroom.

Mohammed is Day 2 and needs the cord clamp removed. I notice they don't yet have a cot or bassinette for the baby – he is sleeping on some small blankets in a plastic oval laundry basket on the floor. In a challenging four-way conversation between two rooms, I complete the necessary tasks of the postnatal visit, and discuss getting a cot from the local Pregnancy Support Service – a great resource for secondhand baby furniture, in-home assistance, clothing and equipment. I show Esra and Hamid a picture of a baby in a cot to reinforce the latest Sudden Infant Death prevention details and arrange for the next visit tomorrow. We organise a time, and I advise I will bring an interpreter again – 'Sorry, not sure of gender, depends on who is available. Hopefully a female . . .'

1200 hours

Shoes on. Outside I thank the interpreter and then the phone rings – it's the special care nursery. Benjamin's blood test from this morning is elevated and he needs to be readmitted for phototherapy treatment. I ask the midwife if she could please contact Jenny and ask her to take Benjamin back to the hospital. I'll see them both later on my return.

1205 hours, 32,307 kilometres
Stuck in the traffic while the train shunts up and down across the main street – time to grab a quick sandwich out of the lunchbox and listen to *Country Hour* on the radio.

1210 hours, 32,307 kilometres
Waiting patiently at the railway line. Get to eat the banana, too – bonus! 'Price of cattle still on the rise . . .'

1225 hours, 32,312 kilometres
'Hello, I'm Jamal. You must be Lyn. Come in – we've been expecting you for lunch.' (Were they really? News to me!) Hardly starving, but not wanting to turn down their hospitality, I say: 'Thank you, but just a small serve, please. I'm on a diet.' I'm shown to the dining room where I'm introduced to Jamal's wife Renata, and her mother, who is busy stirring a big pot of soup on the stove. The table is set, and hot crusty bread rolls are on a plate in the centre. Over a bowl of delicious meat and vegetable broth, we chat about their life in Australia since they settled here from Fiji. Intricate carvings and shell decorations adorn the living area.

Jamal is understandably proud of his firstborn – a son, Anton, now five days old, named after the attending obstetrician. A big baby, weighing almost 4 kilograms. I check Renata out after lunch and her episiotomy is tender – healing well, though.

She's having trouble doing the pelvic floor postnatal exercises and with bladder control. We chat about the exercise techniques and also discuss a referral to the hospital physiotherapist for assessment and ongoing management. Renata agrees to this, and it's arranged that the maternal and child health nurse will visit tomorrow. I thank them for their Polynesian hospitality and wish them well with Anton.

As for the obstetrician – he's invited around for tea tonight!

1345 hours, 32,332 kilometres

The fluids are catching up with me – toilet stop and leg stretch at the local Lions Park.

1350 hours, 32,333 kilometres

Jessica opens the door with tears in her eyes. 'I've had a terrible time since coming home. My nipples are sore and the baby just cries all the time. She was alright in hospital yesterday.'

I know it's going to be a long visit. Jessica is seventeen and this is her first baby. She still lives at home with her parents, who are happy to help. Her dad is at work and her mum has gone shopping. Jessica discloses that the father of the baby had 'long gone' off the scene and wasn't supportive. Baby Shania is four days old and ready for a feed. Jessica has plenty of milk and is obviously struggling to get the baby correctly attached.

I dash out to the car and get the hand breast pump. In a few short minutes, as I nurse a crying Shania, Jessica expresses 30 millilitres of milk. I supervise the baby's positioning and attachment at the breast and observe her sucking action.

'That feels much better – it doesn't hurt near as much,' says Jessica. We sit and talk about the pregnancy and delivery, while Shania has her afternoon tea.

'Grandma' comes home and puts the kettle on and we share a cuppa while Shania continues to feed. She empties one breast well and drifts off to sleep. We discuss all things relevant to breastfeeding and also about booking in tomorrow to the lactation day stay (LDS) clinic. Jessica's mum could drive her the 25 kilometres up to town if they have a vacancy. I give the lactation consultant a call – she could fit her in for the next day, due to a cancellation. I tell Jessica she can borrow the hand pump overnight and I'll collect it tomorrow at the LDS clinic. I leave Jessica with words of encouragement – keep up the fantastic work, good luck with the breastfeeding. She is smiling as I leave . . .

1505 hours, 32,343 kilometres

There are blue balloons on the farm gate. I must be nearly there. Can't see the house. It must be down the tree-lined track and over the rise. Yes, we're here. The blue heeler and the kelpie run out to meet me.

'Don't mind them, they won't bite,' Jack yells out from the shed. I step out of the car dubiously, as Helen opens the front door. From previous experience, I have learned never to trust a blue heeler. I keep my eyes on her, just in case she decides to go for my ankles. Friendly Jess the kelpie is okay, but she jumps up on my skirt with her muddy paws and drags them straight down through my pantyhose. Luckily, it's the last call for the day.

Helen and toddler Jamie usher me inside. Jamie is a bit out of sorts – he's just woken up from his afternoon nap and wonders what all the fuss is about with this new baby brother stuff. He points to the bassinette: 'That's Andoo, and he cries.'

Helen reassures him that baby Andrew is here for keeps and no, the midwife isn't taking him back to the hospital today. Jack comes in to say hello and takes Jamie out to the shed to save me from the 'hundred quick questions' and to give Helen and me a chance to talk.

She recalls that after a long labour and an emergency Caesarean section last time, she attempted to breastfeed but ran into 'all sorts of trouble' in the first week and put Jamie on the bottle. Then she developed postnatal depression by the time he was eight weeks old. Jack really struggled with the concept of her depression and wondered why she couldn't just 'get her act together'.

Fortunately, with medication and good assistance from her local doctor, other family, friends and the local Post & Ante-Natal Depression Association (PANDA) support group, she made a good recovery. Nonetheless, she's quite anxious that it could happen again.

We chat about the circumstances this time around – planned pregnancy, normal delivery, no attempt to breastfeed this time (happy to put Andrew on the bottle from the word go) fewer financial worries, and more confident in all aspects of infant care. All this is reassuring for Helen.

Andrew is just starting to stir. Helen undresses him as the boys come back in from the shed. I weigh and check him out.

'Well done – he's gained 100 grams in two days. The maternal and child health nurse is visiting later on in the week, but give us a call if you have any concerns before then.'

A happy mouse stamp for Andrew's *Child Health Record* book . . . and one for Jamie's forearm.

The black clouds are rolling in and it's just starting to rain as Jack carries the baby scales out to the boot of the car for me. 'Watch out for the kangaroos. The mailman hit one on the way out yesterday in the bush, before he got back to the main road. Wrote his car off!'

With those words of encouragement, I make my way cautiously up the track.

1620 hours, 32,393 kilometres

Back to the car park, wound swab to Pathology, book the interpreter, and Physiotherapy referral to Allied Health before they close. Pick up the new referrals from the maternity ward; turn over the sign to: 'Domiciliary Midwife is In'.

Quick visit to all the Day 2 mums to let them know about our service. Must catch up with Benjamin in the special care nursery. I get an update from his mother, Jenny: yes, he's doing fine with his treatment under the lights.

1705 hours

Off late again, but not always easy to run to a strict schedule. I reflect upon my day as a district midwife. It's an enormous privilege to be invited into the homes of all these interesting people from diverse cultures, socio-economic backgrounds and lifestyles.

'Homes' – now that's another story. Houses, units, caravans, tents, fruit-pickers' huts, renovated churches, buses, backs of shops or factories.

Regardless of where they live, and the signs they use to indicate they are welcoming a new family member, they are all individual people with their own beliefs and personalities. With their lives enriched now that the new baby has arrived, 'home' will never be quite the same again.

Based on true accounts, with names changed and situations altered to protect confidentiality.

MEMORIES, CHANGES and MIRACLES

I'm dancing as fast as I can

BROOKE McREYNOLDS

I don't consider myself old, but changes in midwifery are happening so rapidly that it doesn't take long to fall out of step. Even those of us who recognise progress as positive and who can appreciate the dynamics of development may still, on occasion, find themselves holding the bathwater, wondering what happened to the baby.

The birthing stool was my own personal nemesis.

I had watched films of women giving birth on stools, seemingly effortlessly. Once, while touring another women's hospital, I had come face-to-face with one of these contraptions. This one had resembled a hybrid of a physio table crossed with a shower chair, and no one there that day had actually seen it in use.

Still, I was willing to remain open-minded. What

finally appeared in our own birthing unit looked more like a toddler's training potty. The user was expected to hover over what looked like a tin plate from a mining sluice. I pictured myself in a crouch, with my soon-to-be arthritic knees pressed to the lino and my neck twisted sharply, trying to get a glimpse of the presenting part. 'Can someone please show me how this works?' I said mournfully, seeing myself as Midwife Quasimodo.

'It's easy. I'll show you,' several colleagues reassured me, but I received no actual training before the fateful night when Melissa, one of the young midwives, asked me to fill in for her for five minutes during a labour while she had a quick break. I agreed, happy to stand unobtrusively at the back of the room, alert for disaster but uninvolved.

'She wants to push, but she's got plenty of time,' Melissa called in parting as she closed the door behind her.

Those words made me nervous, so I moved closer to the action.

Mum was seated on the birthing stool near the end of the bed, close enough to lean over the mattress if she wanted to. She, the CTG machine (baby monitor) and the bedside table piled high with drinks, munchies and massage oils, formed a semicircle on one side of the bed. In the centre was a large birthing ball. Who is meant to sit on this, I wondered?

Mum's next contraction was accompanied by a telltale grunt, so I decided to enter the circle, even if only to press the buzzer and summon Melissa back. I struggled with the ball, trying to get someone to help me move it out of the way.

'Melissa sat on the ball,' the family said.

'Sorry, I can't sit on balls,' I said.

'Melissa sat on the ball,' they repeated, fixing me with cold stares. Obviously they had no intention of changing their birth plan for me, despite our 30 seconds of bonding.

So I sat on the ball, tumbling backwards into the bedside table and spilling scented oil down my neck. As my scrambling feet tried to find purchase with the floor, Mum gave another grunt and, peering through my glasses, I saw a large head come into view.

'Don't push! Pant! Pant!' I cried as I pulled on gloves and rolled to the side, cracking my head against the CTG machine. Mum was beyond taking advice from someone she didn't even know, and continued to push. Diving forward, I flew off the ball, banged my chin against her knee and caught the baby by his arm just before he hit the pan.

With blood dribbling from my split lip, I held him aloft triumphantly and steadied myself against the bed with my other hand, not wanting to fall headlong into the dish.

Mum had no intention of accepting this baby from a complete stranger, and as he was still attached to her, I couldn't hand him across the bed to any receptive family members. Draping him over her knee, I cut the cord and gave him to someone with a warm blanket.

I was still trapped by the ball and trying to wriggle around so that I could manoeuvre it out of the way when the placenta landed in the pan with a splat that sprayed me with more blood and liquor. Just then

Melissa waltzed back in, complaining that I had stolen her delivery.

'It wasn't so much stolen as thrust upon me!' I retorted, as the family thanked her for the wonderful job she had done.

Soon after, I was working a night shift and had the opportunity to adapt the birthing stool to me as I had been forced to adapt to it. That night I was also struggling with yet another innovation – the double bed squeezed into the narrow labour room. The bed wasn't adjustable, and at a mid-thigh height, was ideal for dislocating the backs of caregivers.

When Lisa came in to have her baby I happened to be the free midwife and that was the free room. There was no problem at first. Lisa's family, or 'support team' of three, were ready for action. But husband, mother and mother-in-law felt uncomfortable inside the hospital, so they all sat outdoors, with Lisa coming in occasionally for status checks. By the time she was in transition, though, hubby was fast asleep on the double bed, and Shirl and Dot, the mothers, had curled up to sleep in the waiting room.

'Wake us when it's time,' they instructed us.

Back in the room, the nitrous oxide gas was on the far wall, only 30 centimetres from the bed but access was blocked by the baby heater and resuscitation trolley. Since the nitrous hose wasn't long enough to reach the near side of the bed, Lisa had to climb over her slumbering husband to stand between the bed and the wall each time she wanted to use it. She soon gave that away.

When the second stage began, we were finally able to wake hubby and send him off to get the mothers. Then he climbed back on to the double bed so that he could watch in comfort.

With the first good pushing contraction, Shirl fell into Dot's arms, screaming: 'I can't look!'

She wasn't going to leave the room, however, if the other grandmother was staying, so we positioned a chair near the foot of the bed facing the door, so that she could be present without actually watching. Thereafter, with each contraction, she would cry: 'Is it out yet?'

'Not this time,' Dot would answer, pacing up and down.

Shirl would turn around to see for herself, scream, 'I can't watch!' again, and turn back.

Grandmothers sorted, I was having my own problems. As the contractions increased in intensity, Lisa was using motion to help herself cope – by rolling across that large bed.

Call me old-fashioned, but when I am about to deliver a baby I prefer to have the bulging perineum within reach. Lisa's wasn't. I had to figure out a way to keep her near me.

Because I like to offer women choices, I'd offered her the birth stool earlier in the evening, but she preferred the bed, being tired out from having spent the night looking after her support people. The stool now sat in the corner of the room.

With a flash of inspiration, I grabbed it. I placed it in the middle of the bed and coaxed her to sit on it, promising a quicker delivery. Hubby knelt on one side and I was on the other. With Mum and midwife centred, grandmothers providing a cheering section and hubby too gobsmacked to speak, we delivered a beautiful baby boy.

Was this birth because of, or in spite of, my efforts to adapt to new methods? I'll never know.

Look, it's cods!

CAROL MORTON

In 1979, I began my midwifery training in a large hospital in Essex, England. I was really enjoying the course. After a brief spell allocated to the postnatal ward I started an eight-week stint in the antenatal ward.

An old building that many years before had been an isolation hospital, the maternity unit was set up in ancient 'Nightingale'-style wards, a long narrow room with beds running up each side. Big semicircular dayrooms, with glass walls to take advantage of the sunlight, were located at each end of the wards, their bay windows jutting out to overlook the peaceful green landscaped grounds; legacies of the treatment areas for TB patients. Beyond these dayrooms were two smaller rooms, each holding six beds, and used for those patients needing quiet.

Typically, the mums-to-be with no serious medical or obstetric problems were admitted into these smaller rooms to get some 'rest', and it was these patients who usually had the junior student midwives allocated to their care.

On one early shift I was given the task of assessing Mrs Stevens. She had been admitted for 'rest' at 30 weeks gestation with her second pregnancy, and was expecting twins.

My initial assessment included monitoring the two foetal hearts. In those days we used a Pinards stethoscope in conjunction with a handheld Doptone microphone, and I easily located the first heartbeat after palpating and asking Mrs Stevens the usual position of the babies.

The second was harder. Palpation suggested a position that differed from Mrs Stevens' directions. I listened, and sure enough, I heard the second heartbeat, slightly different from that of its sibling.

I was keen to show off my newly acquired knowledge on the subject of foetal monitoring and explained that heartbeats could be heard through the baby's back or abdomen. I began to demonstrate, using the Doptone to pick up the first twin's heart. I explained that, by counting and listening to the pattern of the heartbeat, I could differentiate this baby from the other. I then put the Doptone into the second position to demonstrate the slight variation.

Finally, I put the microphone in the position indicated by Mrs Stevens to show her that it was the same baby. To my astonishment the rate was clearly quite different again! Mrs Stevens had listened to all this, and understandably now became both concerned and confused.

I palpated again, but I wasn't really experienced enough to confirm my mounting belief that Mrs Stevens was carrying not two babies, but three!

I went to the ward sister's office with my charts and information, feeling very excited. I expected some praise, but was met instead with anger and criticism. 'Are you aware of your professional responsibilities to your colleagues?' the ward sister snapped, in mounting fury. 'What makes you such an expert on your very first allocation? How dare you question the competence of others wiser and more experienced than you?'

This last part of her attack was delivered with the wagging finger pointing at my face.

With the final shot of 'Wait until the school hears of this. You'll be lucky not to be sacked!' ringing in my ears, the sister proceeded to make a telephone call to the obstetrician, Mr Deacon. She told him of my impertinence, saying that I had upset the mother-to-be through my inexperience and incompetence when she should have been resting. Finally, she requested that he come and reassure Mrs Stevens himself.

Clearly, Mr Deacon was quite inconvenienced, and I knew that he would expect me to hear his displeasure. He was renowned for reducing nursing staff to tears with his acid tongue.

Further phone calls to the midwifery school and to the director of midwifery resulted in an interview. An 'Adverse Report' was issued to me for causing 'undue stress' to a patient by suggesting a diagnosis that clearly my training hadn't yet enabled me to make.

All of this took place even before Mr Deacon arrived to 'undo the harm' my 'incompetence' had caused.

When Mr Deacon eventually did arrive, I was directed to accompany him, the ward sister and the midwifery school tutor to Mrs Stevens' bedside. The ward sister began by apologising for the student midwife, 'who is very inexperienced still', and then Mr Deacon examined his patient. Using a Pinards stethoscope, he listened to the heartbeats. He palpated and listened again, then he assured Mrs Stevens that everything would be sorted out by an abdominal X-ray. (In the UK in 1979, the use of ultrasound in late pregnancy wasn't common, although every pregnancy was 'scanned' in the first trimester and at the start of the second trimester. After about 28 weeks, however, an abdominal X-ray was the preferred diagnostic aid. This was also routinely undertaken as late as at the onset of labour to diagnose any cephalopelvic disproportion and to confirm the position of babies in a multiple pregnancy. Twins and breech presentations were generally automatically allowed to labour. This usually resulted in successful vaginal deliveries if there was no disproportion between the baby's head and the woman's pelvic size.)

I was taken next to the office in the school of midwifery where my actions were reviewed. I was asked to explain why I, a student midwife, thought I should question a diagnosis. After all, the senior tutor continued, there had been a number of doctors and experienced midwives involved in the care of Mrs Stevens during the 30 weeks of her pregnancy so far, and no one else had questioned the number of babies she was carrying.

By the time I returned to the ward, I felt like a wrung-out dishrag. At last, the ward sister sent me to the staff room for a break. There I had more explaining to do to the various staff members, who had heard all about this 'jumped-up little upstart' who thought she knew everything. This was a perfect example of a hospital 'grapevine' at work.

Later on that shift, Mrs Stevens returned from the X-ray department with the results of her abdominal X-ray and pelvimetry. Mr Deacon was right; the X-ray really did confirm the diagnosis.

FOUR babies showed up clearly, all arrayed in a line. Four breech presentations.

I never did get a formal apology, but the 'Adverse Report' was withdrawn from my personal records.

For weeks this story was the talk of the hospital, as there had never been quads delivered there before.

I was certainly not treated any differently on the wards or by my fellow students, but I did have one of the midwifery tutors congratulate me on 'sticking to my guns' despite the hostile reaction by the senior staff.

Later in my training, when the midwifery tutors covered the topic of 'professional accountability', this actual incident was used as an example of how to resolve conflicting diagnoses.

Mr Deacon continued to look after Mrs Stevens, who had a Caesarian three weeks later. By that time, my eight-week rotation on the antenatal ward had ended and I was working in the neonatal intensive-care nursery.

The best thing to come from this incident was that Mrs Stevens specifically requested that I be involved in her delivery. I was the only student midwife in the elite team assembled to attend this auspicious moment in the history of the maternity unit.

I was asked by no less a personage than Mr Deacon himself to be one of the four midwives chosen to work with a paediatrician forming four teams. The midwife would 'receive' each baby from the surgeon as it was delivered and carry it to the resuscitation trolly where the paediatrician waited. When I was asked which baby I wanted to be responsible for, I chose to 'receive' baby number three. Only the midwife and the paediatrician team involved with the third baby would be actually present in the theatre for all four deliveries, and I wanted to see all four born.

The three girls and one boy were all born healthy and vigorous. All were admitted to the neonatal intensive-care unit but really required little more than transient care.

The local paper later ran a picture of the older brother, two-year-old Christopher, standing over the four lustily crying babies who were all lined up, with the caption: 'Look, it's CODS!' (He couldn't say 'quads'.)

For a few years afterwards I kept in contact with the Stevens family. Each time they visited the hospital they would phone to arrange to bring the quads to see us, and I also attended their first birthday party. The nickname 'CODS' stuck firmly to the four for about a year.

In 2000 the local newspaper carried a picture of them at 21 years of age using the same caption. There was a brief story about the surprise of their birth, but no mention of me or of the way Mrs Stevens' expected babies doubled in number.

Separated at birth

CHRISTINE CROYDEN

Friday afternoon and the labour ward was buzzing. Babies were crying behind closed doors and midwives rushed about, wheeling trolleys and pushing cots and equipment from room to room. I hung up my cape and paused; the next eight hours were not going to be dull. In the office, medical students were being shooed out in preparation for the arrival of the charge midwife, Caroline Carr. She was outside room 2 deep in conversation with a middle-aged woman who could have come straight from the races in her tailored red suit, matching hat and high-heeled patent leather shoes. Caroline looked at the clock and towards us through the office window as we waited for her to come and allocate our patients.

We watched with interest as the woman spoke

intensely into Caroline's face and used her hands to drive home each point she made. Intermittently, she would gesture towards room 2, in a frantic, desperate way, as if whatever was going on in there was unacceptable. Eventually they reached an agreement and Caroline extended her hand to the woman who hesitated, then shook it briefly. Neither seemed happy with the outcome, and when the woman smiled politely at Caroline it was a manufactured smile that didn't reach her eyes.

Caroline walked briskly back into the office, her lips pursed tightly and her heavy brows knitted in a frown that she usually reserved only for errant medical students. The woman glanced across at me through the window: she'd seen me staring at her and wasn't happy about it. I looked down at my shoes as she slipped back into room 2.

For the change of shift handover I'd wedged myself in the corner between several of my colleagues with the hope of remaining inconspicuous. We all waited in silence as Caroline looked critically at the patient names on the white board in front of her and then around the room at us. Her gaze stopped at me and I straightened up, knocking a clipboard off the desk and on to the floor. 'How many deliveries do you need to make your 25?' she asked.

'Only three.'

'Okay,' she said, folding her arms. 'There's a young girl in room 2. She's sixteen and about 36 weeks gestation – but we can't be sure because the mother hasn't managed to get her to one antenatal appointment. Anyway, it looks like she's posterior. She ruptured her membranes during a maths class and has come here straight from school. I'd hazard a guess that she'll deliver before lunch.'

I swallowed hard and felt around in my pockets for my pens and fob watch.

'Lynne's in there. She'll supervise. You do the delivery.'

I went to take the girl's notes and as Caroline passed them across the crowded room she added gently, 'Make sure you do exactly what Lynne tells you to.'

Not bloody Lynne. I'd sat next to her in the cafeteria the night before and listened quietly as she demolished the character of one of my friends to another labour ward midwife – who was also a well-known dragon. The competence of anyone trained in Australia was the gist of the conversation. They both hailed from Edinburgh and were particularly appalled by the poor quality of students in my intake of novice midwives, whom they agreed were the worst lot they'd had to put up with for years.

I walked into room 2 and closed the door carefully. A girl wearing her school socks and a white hospital gown writhed on the bed. Her blazer was draped over a chair, and a bag covered with U2 stickers and drawings of large coloured hearts with names written inside them was on the floor in the corner. By the window, looking out on to Lonsdale Street, stood the woman, who had removed her hat and jacket to reveal a pristine white shirt and ropes of pearls. Her arms were folded and her fists clenched tightly, but her face was blank when she looked in my direction as I entered the room.

'Okay, so you're here. Go and set up your trolley. It

won't be long,' Lynne said with her back to me as she struggled to put a roll of paper into the new foetal monitor. I went over to the bed.

'I'm going to help you deliver your baby, Sarah,' I said. She looked up with an expression of terror mixed with a sort of incomprehension that I'd only seen on children's faces when they were being yelled at for something they didn't know they'd done. 'But I need you to help,' I added, touching her arm.

'Just HURRY,' she sobbed. Her face was puffy and swollen from crying. I could feel Lynne's breath on the back of my neck.

'Where's your trolley? Scrub up, she's in transition . . . and hurry. We don't have time for you to mess around,' Lynne said harshly as she prised the girl's knees apart and stared between her legs. 'Wait,' she said to her firmly. 'Don't you push yet.'

'Get it out,' the girl screamed, looking across at her mother standing frozen by the window. I scrubbed up quickly and pulled on my gloves and then walked towards the bed with my hands in the air. Lynne nodded her head impatiently. 'Well, get in there. You know what to do,' she commanded.

I bent forward just as another contraction gripped the girl. 'Okay, Sarah. Now PUSH,' I said loudly in an attempt to rein in her focus. She was trying hard, but shaking and crying had made her lose control halfway through the pain.

'Try again, Sarah . . . as soon as the next one starts,' I said, looking at her directly with my elbows keeping her trembling legs apart. Lynne stood opposite me holding the girl's slim thighs just below the drapes so as to pin her pelvis to the bed. A contraction began and Sarah's perineum blanched white.

'That's right. They're a lot easier to get in than they are to get out,' Lynne muttered.

I looked up at her face, which was inches from mine. Without missing a beat, she asked: 'How many episiotomies have you cut?'

'Only one.'

'Well, you're going to cut another one now.'

Here we go. I felt myself starting to sweat.

'Pick up your scissors and tell me how you're going to cut.'

'At a 45-degree angle.'

'Do it now. She's going to tear.'

I put my scissors in position and with one hand firmly over the baby's crowning head cut hard through the stretched white skin and muscle. The head sprang out and blood spurted over us both. Sarah let out one almighty scream, pushed again and her baby slid out. A girl.

'Wrap her up and take her out of here. I'll deliver the placenta,' Lynne said, barely giving me time to cut the cord as she pushed in front of me.

'But . . .' I said, picking up the baby.

The woman in the corner walked over to us. 'She doesn't want to see the baby . . .' she whispered. 'Just take it out now, please, dear.'

'She's perfect. Can't she hold her?' I said, wiping the baby's round face and positioning her in the crook of my arm for her grandmother to see how vigorously she could kick.

She looked away. 'NO, she can't. Just do as I ask, NOW.'

I stopped for a moment and looked at Sarah, who'd slumped back on to her bloodied sheets. She was staring up at the ceiling as Lynne delivered the placenta, which plopped out between her legs, barely causing her to stir. Lynne laid it on the bed beside the girl and began to run her gloved hands over the shiny surface to check that it was all there.

Sarah glanced down at the red blob briefly, then beyond the window glass into the distant sky. Perhaps she was forever fixing this moment of her life into her memory – layer upon layer of tightly packed images – or maybe she was trying to block them out.

I wrapped the baby up and took her over to Lynne, who grunted dismissively and nudged me closer towards the door with her hip. I hesitated, then turned the knob slowly and walked into the corridor where the air was thinner and cooler. I stood with my back against the closed door and pressed the baby's little body to mine. Her fist was partly in her mouth and her navy blue eyes were wide open and looking up at me.

I waited there, shaking with her in my arms, then as I shifted my gaze up from the baby's face I saw Caroline Carr watching us through the window from her desk. For a moment I held the baby more tightly and thought about taking her back inside to her mother. Caroline shook her head, almost imperceptibly, and began rifling about on her desk. She quickly found what she was looking for and stood before me holding up a document. It looked like signed adoption papers.

Suddenly I became aware of voices and faces and trolleys rushing past, and of the bright, fluorescent lights beaming down on us both. I walked towards the nursery and placed the baby into a clean, warm cot ready to begin my routine newborn check.

Names and some details have been changed to protect confidentiality.

Weekend guest

LEE PATTINSON

Not for the first time, Nell blessed the person who had thought to add a small deck to the rear of the health centre's flat. It caught the morning sun and was a perfect spot for a peaceful breakfast. She stretched lazily, finished the last of the tea in her cup.

An easy day today – half-day at Toonbridge, then home visits, with only three scheduled.

Two of them should be easy, one no more than a courtesy call on a family recently moved down here from Caulfield. She'd had the referral card and summary of the history, which showed the mother had visited regularly and appeared to have no problems.

The second call would be the last she'd be making to Mrs Belmont, who would be coming in to the clinic after this week. The third visit was the only one that might take a little time – Mrs Gibson, discharged from the local hospital this week with her baby girl.

Matron Arnold had expressed concern about her. 'Might have to settle for a bottle there,' she'd said. 'Mum's not producing, even with demand feeding and expressing. They might settle down when they get home, but I wouldn't count on it.'

Nell had known Jenny Arnold since their midwifery training days. It was Jenny who had convinced her to move to Woodford to take over the centre ten years before. Best thing any friend had ever done for her. Nell was content here in this little town where everything was within walking distance, everyone smiled at everyone else in the street, even at visiting strangers. The hospital was equipped to deal with all but the most serious of cases, and they had a helicopter on call for those. In the 1950s the RAAF had retired surplus Second World War aircraft to civilian medical use, a welcome blessing for country areas. The arrival of one was an event watched by the entire town.

Best of all, the town had Dr Keith Rawlings, who might have stepped from the pages of a novel describing the perfect country medico. He'd been running his solo practice here for over twenty years and by now it was almost his own private hospital. The board trusted him to make all the medical decisions without question – and fortunately, he'd never made a wrong one in all the years he'd been there. He knew every patient by their first name, was doing second-generation deliveries for many families, and would turn out of bed at any hour of the day or night when called on.

Nell couldn't believe her luck when she compared him

with some of the doctors other centre sisters had to deal with. Dr Rawlings, once satisfied she knew her job, left her to get on with it. One of her most treasured moments was when a mother came for a weaning program saying, 'I went to Dr Rawlings and he shot me off here. Said you'd forgotten more about that than he'd ever known, so you were the expert.'

As she had expected, Toonbridge was quiet, with only half-a-dozen mothers coming in, one of them with the latest addition to the Penfold household. Nell smiled to herself as she remembered Dr Rawlings' warning about them. 'Don't ask too closely about parentage when you fill out their forms,' he'd said with a grin. 'Three brothers, all fishermen, all away at different times but seeing that one of them's always at home to look after things. More than just household repairs, I gather, so goodness knows who fathers who. But the kids are well-cared-for and flourishing, better than a lot of other kids around here, so who are we to find fault?'

The last mother gone, Nell ate a sandwich, poured coffee from her thermos and got ready for her visiting. As anticipated, two of the calls were dealt with quickly and it was still early as she headed out along the road through the Soldier Settlement blocks, government-allocated housing for returned servicemen. The Gibson farm was one of them.

The road to the Prom was smooth and cared for – thank goodness for tourists! The names of the owners were on their mailboxes, so finding the Gibson place was easy. Not like some first visits she had made, when she had spent plenty of time and petrol trying to find a property concealed in the hills.

She parked in front of the small weatherboard house and knew what she was going to find inside it – the wails of a baby in distress came loudly through the open front door. Pamela Gibson was already opening the flywire door and stepping out before Nell even had her car door open – 'Oh, thank goodness you've come, Sister. I can't get her to stop crying!' she said, distraught.

She had the shawl-wrapped baby over one shoulder and was patting ineffectually at the small heaving back. Nell quickly put her bag down on a small table on the verandah and reached for the baby. With practised hands she loosened the wrappings, and wasn't surprised to see the baby's knees jerk to a point almost under her chin as soon as the restraints were gone. Quickly she elicited a history of events.

'Well, she always seems hungry. But when I give her a bit more of the bottle, she takes it then starts crying again and usually brings some back up . . .' Nell was relieved to hear that it wasn't projectile vomiting. 'And she hardly sleeps at all, except for maybe half an hour or so when she's completely worn out. I didn't have much breast-milk in the hospital and it's gone altogether now; I think it's because I haven't been getting any sleep either.'

A few more questions and Nell knew that her initial guess was almost certainly right – this was a classic case of severe colic, quite possibly due to a cow's milk allergy.

Jim, the young father, had come in and he looked at Nell with an expression of utter astonishment. 'You mean to say I've got a herd of pure-bred Jerseys right at the back door and she can't take milk? Don't reckon I'm too keen on getting any of that powdered crap in tins from the chemist when I've got better stuff right here!'

'Well, maybe it won't come to that, Mr Gibson. I'll see if I can find another answer.'

Nell knew that many parents were suspicious of the tins of baby formula that were starting to appear on chemist's shelves and not even the most assiduous advertising campaign could convince them it was better for some babies. Even worse, some firms were promoting diluted sweetened condensed milk – a boon for future dentists, she had once heard that described.

'What do you want us to do?' Mrs Gibson asked anxiously.

Nell answered on impulse. 'Let me have her for the weekend – would you do that?'

It was obviously a totally unexpected answer and the parents exchanged startled looks.

'I'll take great care of her and it will give me a chance to see how the attacks come in relation to other events – feeding, nappy changes and so forth . . .'

'Oh, we're not worried about you looking after her properly, Sister. It just seems a bit much to ask you to do that.'

'*You're* not asking – *I* am. And the shire pays me to solve parents' problems.'

The young dad switched the baby seat to Nell's car, while Mum packed the necessities: bottles, a supply of teats, nappies, changes of clothing, and a big screw-top jar of their own cow's milk – 'This morning's milking and it's been in the fridge since then.'

Nell made a courtesy call to Dr Rawlings when she got back and apologised for not checking with him beforehand. 'Actually,' she confessed, 'I didn't know I was going to do it until I saw them, and it seemed the right thing to do.'

'They'll think you're an angel in disguise if they get a good night's sleep, Sister,' chuckled the doctor. 'It was probably an act of mercy, if only for that!'

Nell made a call to Jenny to talk the problem over with her, and also spoke with a friend who had a herd of Saanan goats. Then she was ready for the weekend ahead.

At two o'clock the following morning she wasn't quite so sure of the wisdom of her decision. At four o'clock, still sleepless, she was convinced she had been stupid. But things eased off during Saturday daytime hours, and the baby woke up only twice on Saturday night. Then she slept almost all of Sunday – and Nell felt a surge of triumph.

She had arranged for the Gibsons to come in early on Monday, before she opened the centre. She wanted to outline what she had done and what she wanted them to do. They had rung for progress reports during the weekend, of course, and she had assured them they were welcome to stop in at any time if they wanted to reassure themselves that all was well, but she was inwardly pleased they hadn't taken her up on her suggestion.

The first time Pamela Gibson had phoned in to Nell, the baby had been wailing so loudly she'd had to go through to the clinic office to take the call on the extension. Now, both parents looked in disbelief at their baby, cosily wrapped and sleeping soundly in the clinic bassinette.

Pamela whispered: 'That's the very first time I've seen her really sleeping. At home, even when she did drop off for a while, she was still twitching and whimpering all the time, not sleeping peacefully as she is now. I don't know how you did it, Sister!'

'Well,' Jim said resignedly, 'if that's what this chemist stuff does for her, then I'll pay for it, even though I hate passing over good cash for tinned second-best muck!'

'Oh, don't worry too much about that,' smiled Nell. 'I noticed on Friday that you have a nice little herd of goats out there, and a few nannies with kids, so what I've done is weaned her on to goat's milk, which she seems to be able to digest without any problem.'

The young dad was delighted. 'You little beauty, Sis! Never thought about that myself! I reckon a bloke oughta change his will and leave you a thumping great bonus, just for getting us this last three nights' sleep! And seeing to it that there's more to come . . .'

Jenny, a born cynic, sniffed when Nell told her. 'Should have got it in writing on the spot, sucker,' was all she said.

These events happened in the 1960s when I had the health centre in Foster, South Gippsland. Infant formula wasn't in common use, with most babies either being breastfed (with expressed milk from other mums, in some cases) or given diluted cow's milk. Other not-to-be-recommended bottle feedings were made from diluted sweetened condensed milk or diluted evaporated milk.

Queasy rider

SUSAN DEMORAY

There was no consoling Sheila Golightly as she lurched on the tram. She winced. 'Maybe my plan isn't so hot,' she thought. 'Yes, after only a week, it's looking decidedly dodgy!'

She'd lugged a large cardboard box with a hole in it, and a squinty-eyed rag doll on to the tram with her. Pale-faced, pale-lipped young women in orange bum-freezer skirts nudged one another, clicking their tongues at her. Two little boys crooked their fingers suggestively at the box, whistling through the gaps in their teeth. Their ogling stopped when their mother clouted them, and shouted: 'Eh, you! Stupida!'

Sheila screwed up her pancake-powdered face and black-lined eyes at them all. She sighed. 'So, what's happening, then? Midwifery should be easy; it only goes for twelve months!'

Catching the tram was the only way Sheila, a student midwife, could get to the Royal Women's Hospital. She had to go there for training. Somehow. A qualification from this world-renowned hospital would be her meal ticket for overseas travel – her bid for freedom.

The student midwives used boxes and dolls in their birthing tutorials. Only Sheila shoved her box and doll away. 'How can this piece of cardboard represent a woman's pudenda? And this doll! A cuddly new baby? It's so bloody ugly! It looks like a prop for a Hammer horror film!'

The tutor, wearing a Second World War-era starched white veil and a look to match, sniffed at Sheila. 'Pay attention, Golightly! We use this mechanism box to demonstrate how the baby's head rotates in the mother's pelvis. A normal delivery is all about control: keeping control of the baby's head, keeping the crown up. Remember, flex the baby's chin.'

'How the hell do I remember this?' Sheila whispered to Tanya Shultz, an Alfred Hospital graduate. 'I couldn't even remember what went on an enema tray. I always forgot the clamp!'

After a few weeks the tutorials finished, and the student midwives witnessed real births. They fronted up to the newly-designed delivery ward.

'At the Women's we take a modern approach to obstetrics. We have private delivery rooms,' chortled the charge sister. 'A big improvement on our old labour ward. It only had curtains around the beds.'

'We heard about that ward. And the pelvics happening in the bathroom,' muttered Tanya. She loved quoting Karl Marx to Sheila and was a fanatic about procedure. She lectured multigravida mothers on how to breastfeed. And wondered why they hooted with laughter.

Witnessing her first birth, Sheila expected the ultimate in modern procedure. But instead, sprawled on a bed, there was a woman who howled like a banshee. She jerked about on her left side with her upper leg strapped up high to a pole. A midwife stooped behind the woman, with her arm over the heaving abdominal hulk, her hand between the woman's thighs. And Sheila hankered for the box and ugly doll.

Male medical students lounged up against the delivery room wall. They were gawking in their white shirts and pants and prissy white bow-ties. Among them was Oliver Biggitt-Smythe, who she could hang out with, who made her laugh.

Sheila didn't see much of the baby – she won the short straw and scored weighing the placenta. Oliver tracked her into the utility room. He poked the bluish quivering mass in the kidney dish and smirked. 'Wow, let's fire up the barbecue.'

Sheila seized the kidney dish from him. 'A cadaver soufflé would be more your scene!' she sneered. 'What the fuck was all that in the delivery room, Oliver? I mean how easy would it be to push out a baby in that position? And then be forced to flash your arse at a bunch of pubescent blow-ins? No wonder the poor bugger was screeching!'

Oliver straightened his bow-tie. 'The professor says there's more control with a left lateral position. It cuts down perineal tears,' he said.

'Well, how they treat women patients here makes me want to puke!'

'You've forgotten that the patient is Greek.'

'Eh? What do you mean?' she snapped, as she flung the placenta on to the scales.

'Sheila, the charge sister told us to ignore Greek women screaming. In labour, they scream like this all the time. It's their way of scaring off evil spirits. The louder, the better.'

'Yeah? You saying migrant women are primitives?'

He shrugged coldly. Where was the Biggitt-Smythe who used to make her laugh?

Sheila tossed the placenta in the bin, shoved Oliver aside and started to scrub the utility room. Her vigour in such menial tasks was rare. A sense of relief flooded her body as she scrubbed, though, and daydreamed about the film *Easy Rider*. She had argued with Tanya about the Peter Fonda and Dennis Hopper characters. Escaping on Harley-Davidson motorbikes, Peter and Dennis went for the easy ride. And some redneck shot them for it. So, what kind of freedom was that? Tanya declared that two people alone couldn't achieve a revolution.

Months later, it was Sheila's first delivery that seemed revolting. She froze in the delivery room. She could see the baby's head crowning. No rag doll now.

'Go on, take your bloody time, why don't you?' sniggered Sister O'Reilly. She had the eyes of a cornered rhino and the forearms of Popeye. Like a circus knife-thrower, she hurled a pair of scissors at Sheila. 'Snip that perineum, quick! She's going to tear,' she said.

Sheila's hands trembled with the scissors. She felt cold and clammy and wanted to throw up. 'I can't do it!' she cried. 'I can't!'

How would it feel if someone cut me down there! Ugh!

'Ah, you're worse than Bradford!' bawled O'Reilly.

Oh, Sheila knew about Bradford. He was a medical student with a fondness for splitting hairs. On his delivery day he had also revolted. Crossing his arms as his patient was pushing, he announced it just wasn't a good day for a delivery. No one was going to force him to deliver her and that was that! Too bad about that baby's head! Let it crown!

Sheila knew that, like Bradford, she needed twenty deliveries to qualify. But she could never snip away at another woman's perineum! *Never!* It was living flesh, soft with blood in it. It wasn't cardboard!

Immediately, O'Reilly ordered Sheila to assist with an antenatal examination. Outside the patient's room, Sheila heard someone barking: 'Get on the bed, you! Go on!'

Sheila found a young pregnant Italian woman, sobbing away and cowering before a grey-haired man, or doctor, in a grey suit. He frowned at Sheila and grunted as she approached the bed. Then he continued to bellow at the woman until she lay limp on the bed, like a rag doll.

Sheila reeled and left the room, leaving the grey man to it. *Aliens were little grey creatures, too.* Why did this incident deal such a blow, though? Doctors screeched at their patients at her regional hospital, after all. Maybe it was the aura of vulnerability about the young woman, with her swinging gut and Pidgin English.

Sheila wondered if the grey man would report her defiance.

'The hospital will follow procedure,' chattered Tanya excitedly. 'Here, old Grammar boys are the ruling class. So, forget dobbing in that doctor. He might treat women like lab rats, but O'Reilly worships him. The whole place worships him. They say he's made an important medical discovery.'

'I know what he needs to discover,' Sheila muttered. 'Patience.'

Sure enough, over the next few months, reports of Sheila's belligerence surfaced. The hospital noted that Sheila was a student who floundered – one who rivalled Bradford in reputation. And Sheila now knew she was struggling to keep alive her bid to escape.

Then, one day, she felt so loaded in her gut it made her nauseous. The sickbay doctor eyed her suspiciously, like a pig looks at a wok. 'Student midwives don't get sick. They just get pregnant,' he muttered.

'I'm not going to be shot down by this redneck,' she thought.

'Do an examination, then. You'll find I'm not up the duff,' she cried, her face burning. 'I'm in agony. It's this horrible weight in my stomach.'

He peered at his Rolex watch. 'You might just need an enema,' he offered.

'It's your head that needs an enema! And don't forget to clamp it!' she thought, swishing the curtain on her way out.

In her tenth month, Sheila collapsed. The hospital performed emergency surgery and removed ovarian cysts so massive that most of Sheila's 21-year-old ovaries had to go as well. She was told she could not have children.

Be thankful, they said, that these cysts didn't have hair or teeth in them. Matron visited in her starched veil.

'Ah, you have plenty of reading material, Sister,' she said as she picked up Sheila's books – *The Communist Manifesto* and *The Life of Lenin*. Gingerly, she awarded Sheila a tin of sour lemon drops.

Along with her ovaries, Sheila Golightly lost her will.

'I just can't finish training,' she thought. 'Face it; taking my ovaries is a sign I don't belong here. Even Karl Marx would hate his gonads becoming communal property! Is "Liberty a whore" like Peter Fonda said in *Easy Rider*? Or like Tanya says, is my idea of freedom just an opiate of the people?'

Administration sent her to Emergency. To recover. And, there, she tried to figure out her new plans. *What now? Finding eggs on Easter Island?*

Then one night, when the other Emergency staff were at tea, a man smothered in stubble belted into Emergency. 'Quick, Sister, there's a woman out there having a bloody baby!' he shouted.

Sheila wanted to tell the man she wasn't deaf. But his frantic waving stopped her. She bolted after him out of the Emergency door and towards a taxi, parked in the hospital car park. She saw the back door of the taxi flung open. And the taxi-driver melt into the darkness.

The lights in the taxi didn't work and all Sheila could see was a blob on the back seat. It was heaving.

'Hurry up, love!' said the blob. 'The little bugger's nearly here.'

Here she was, alone, in the dark and without equipment, gown or gloves. *Where was everybody? Wouldn't they know she was missing?*

Sheila yelled for help. No one came. Not even the taxi-driver.

'Aw, don't worry, love,' said the blob, who started pushing, her legs splayed along the car seat. 'We don't need nothin'. It'll be a piece of cake.'

'Keep talking,' Sheila replied, trying to sound cheerful. 'I've got to find the right end.'

Sheila found and flexed the baby's chin and felt a little head crowning. She felt the wetness of its hair, and the softness of the emerging head. She felt the sweat and blood of the woman's flesh. She felt the rush of the baby's head as it plunged out into the world. *No cardboard box, no left lateral position, no audience*. Just her, the blob, and the baby ineffably bound as one in those few minutes.

The baby's legs jabbed vigorously. 'It's a girl,' laughed the mother. 'Another one.'

Sheila didn't know whether to laugh or cry. Suddenly everything felt real. She wrapped the baby up in the bottom of the woman's dress and screeched again for help. The taxi-driver stepped from the shadows.

'Over, is it?' he said sheepishly as he stared at Sheila's bloodied hands and uniform.

'Get someone from Emergency! We need baby stuff and a trolley! Move!' Sheila bellowed.

The driver found Mr Burt, an old orderly, and they scurried out dragging a trolley. They wrapped the baby in a warm bunny rug and then loaded the mother and child on to the trolley. Sheila trotted beside them as Mr Burt pushed the trolley back into Emergency. The woman grabbed Sheila's hands, as tears welled up in her eyes.

'Thanks, love,' she said. 'We'll never forget you. What's your name?'

Two days later, Sheila, running late as usual, rushed to the lift. There were medical students with clipboards and prissy white bow-ties prattling about the professor and cold speculums. And there was a huge, dishevelled woman jammed in a wheelchair pushed by Mr Burt. The woman tapped her on the arm and whispered, 'Hi, Sheila.'

Sheila hesitated. She didn't recognise the face.

'I'm Vera Cassidy. From the taxi the other night,' continued the woman, her dull eyes scanning for Sheila's response. 'Oh, and Sheila is doing well, too.'

'Who?' said Sheila, suddenly alert.

'Sheila . . . we named the baby after you. We wouldn't have managed without you!'

Sheila's heavily black-lined eyes suddenly turned to wet patchy blotches, the outer rims vampiric and ecstatic. Tears do that with cheap mascara. At that moment, her struggles at the hospital seemed worth it. She thought: 'Who gives a shit if this midwifery is hard? Or if I stuffed up? I've made up my mind! I'll slog out this last month or so and graduate, damn it!'

Mr Burt parked Vera in the corridor and followed Sheila when she left the lift.

'A word, Sister,' he said, pulling at her elbow, his wizened face creasing into a grin. 'Lived around here all me life, yer know. Seen many changes: those high-rise flats and spaghetti lovers comin' in packs . . .'

'I'm happy for you, Mr Burt. So . . .'

'Some things never change, Sister.'

Sheila looked at him blankly.

'I'm talking about our Vera Cassidy,' he said, still grinning.

'Vera?'

'She lives near me. Yer shouldn't get too chuffed about Vera.'

'What are you on about, Mr Burt?'

'Vera's never had a baby in a hospital. She plans it that way, see. She likes to have 'em her way. And she's had a few.'

Sheila edged closer to the old man. *Was Vera smashed that night?*

'Eh? A few what?' she said.

'A few kids. She's 'ad a few.'

'Oh? How many?'

'Eight she admits to. I could tell yer were feelin' kinda honoured by her namin' the baby after yer. It's not that big a deal for Vera, though. She names each baby after the person who helps her 'ave it.'

Sheila Golightly shifted from one foot to the other and forgot she was late for duty. Bewildered, she nodded at Mr Burt and glanced back at Vera's fatigued face.

Vera's gaze back at her, lit with affection, launched the memory of that moment in the taxi. Instantly, Sheila recognised the remarkable energy that she had shared with Vera and with Sheila Jr. *The three of them had become one extraordinary organism!* The experience had delivered much more than just Vera's baby. Sheila now understood the meaning of togetherness and respect.

'And I don't need Tanya Schultz or Karl Marx to tell me how it should be,' she mused.

From then on, the memory of that experience was like a newborn of her own.

Drawing its first breath.

Sheila Golightly was me. After graduation I went overseas as planned and had many on-road adventures – a bit like Peter Fonda and Dennis Hopper. But, happily, my ride was far easier and lasted much longer.

Sarah

DIANNE BOSHAMMER

I started my midwifery training in 1985 and, like many of my colleagues, was young and very inexperienced in everything relating to babies. Of course, I had nieces and nephews and had watched them grow up, but I had never been really touched by the impact that a baby like Sarah could make on my life.

Melissa was a trainee nurse. I had seen her many times in the hospital canteen lined up like the rest of us for meals but had never really gotten to know her. Through the hospital grapevine I had heard she was pregnant. This really interested me for several reasons. As a young woman myself, childless and I suppose a little 'green', I found myself wondering what it was like for her. What would it be like to be eighteen and pregnant? Did she have a partner? Was she going to give up her career in nursing?

One day at morning tea Melissa came and sat with us, the lowly student midwives. She looked tired and drawn and like she needed to be anywhere but at work.

'You look beat,' said Mary, one of the youngest midwives.

'I am,' sighed Melissa. 'I just want to be in bed resting.'

'So, are you going to have this baby?' blurted Anne, a midwife who was never afraid to ask the questions we were all thinking.

'Yes,' said Melissa. 'I don't believe in abortion. Just because I made a silly mistake doesn't mean I'm not going to go through with it.'

'You're braver than me, Sunshine,' said Louise, between mouthfuls of her coffee.

Melissa smiled sadly. 'I don't think I'm brave. I'm just doing what I think is best for the baby. I don't plan to keep it. I plan to carry this baby, give birth and then hand it over to someone I know will give him or her everything I can't. I've spoken to the matron and she is organising for me to have time off work and to restart my training three months after the baby is born.'

We all looked at each other in total disbelief. Had she really thought this through?

Over the next few months I occasionally saw Melissa in the canteen looking more and more pregnant, and although I never got to speak to her again, I often wondered how she was feeling. Eventually she left the hospital and went home to her parents to wait for the birth. She had mentioned that her parents had been very supportive of her decision not only to continue with the pregnancy but also to adopt the baby out.

During her pregnancy Melissa had seen a counsellor and talked about her adoption plans and how she had decided she wasn't ready to become a mother yet. She wanted this child to have more than she could offer at this time of her life and career. The counsellor had talked to her about how hard it would be. She was told she would have 30 days after the birth to think about it.

Sarah's birth-day came one fine spring morning. Melissa was at full term and more than ready physically to give birth. Her mother, Betty, had offered to be her support person during labour. She held Melissa's hand and carried her bag as together they walked into the maternity unit. The contractions were coming frequently and painfully.

The labour was long and arduous. It was a journey that Melissa had read about but, like all first labours, didn't really know what she was in for. Betty helped her as much as she could, rubbing her daughter's back and offering her hand while Melissa squeezed it hard during the strong contractions.

'I can't do this anymore, Mum,' Melissa wept.

'Yes you can,' soothed her mother. 'I'm here and I can help. You're not alone, honey.'

Finally, late that night, the time came. Betty held Melissa's hand while she bore down. Mary, the student midwife on duty, stood in anticipation and murmured gentle words of encouragement as the baby's head crowned. This was to be Mary's first unassisted birth. The senior labour midwife, Alice, stood on the opposite side of the bed ready to help if Mary needed it.

'Gently does it, Mary,' she advised as the head emerged. 'Just breathe now, Melissa. No more pushing.'

Mary quickly checked to see if the cord was around the baby's neck, then the body slipped out with a rush. Mary lifted Sarah up on to Melissa's chest. 'It's a girl!' she exclaimed, as she cut the cord to separate mother and child.

Melissa held Sarah, who was covered in vernix and a little blood, and looked deep into her eyes. *Could* she be a mother? *Could* she give up everything she wanted to care for this child? Betty had tears in her eyes as she kissed Melissa ever so gently on the cheek.

'She is so beautiful,' she murmured, as Melissa cried tears of relief and joy.

Mary stood close by triumphantly – she had done it, and all had gone well. She, too, was crying. Alice had been involved with many births where the child was to be given up for adoption. She gently said to Melissa: 'She needs to go now.'

Sarah cried and was lifted off Melissa's chest and taken to the nursery to be weighed, bathed and fed. Her life as an 'adoptive' baby had just begun.

Adoption was quite the norm in 1985 and until the early 1990s. There could be up to two or three babies a month waiting for adoption and these babies would be cared for in the nursery by the midwives. Some of us were mothers ourselves, the rest of us were childless and inexperienced. Here the baby stayed until their mother had signed the adoption papers and the new parents had viewed the baby and been interviewed for their suitability. This could be quite a lengthy process and in Sarah's case took over six weeks. It was unusual that a baby stayed longer than four weeks in the nursery. Foster parents were fairly uncommon in 1985, and they rarely looked after a baby who was up for adoption.

While Sarah was being settled into the nursery, Melissa was taken to the postnatal unit. Her bed was in the corner, well away from the nursery and the other mothers and their babies. I was on duty when Melissa came into the ward. She was exhausted and yet had such a radiant look on her face.

'Hi, there,' I said as she was gently lifted on to her bed from the steel trolley. 'How are you feeling?'

'Absolutely exhausted,' she replied.

'Sleep now,' I said. 'I'll try not to disturb you too often. I just need to do some observations, feel your fundus and check your loss. Is that okay?'

'Sure,' she said as she fell asleep.

Later that night, Melissa awoke feeling much more rested.

'How are you now?' I asked and pulled a chair up beside her bed to sit and have a chat with her.

'Better, thanks,' she replied as she sat up in bed and brushed her hair from her face. Then the questions tumbled out in quick succession. 'What is she like?' she asked. 'Does she look like me? How heavy is she?'

'She is beautiful,' I replied. 'She is 7 pound 3 ounces. I don't know if she looks like you, sorry. I really haven't been able to have a good close look at her.'

'What's her name?' asked Melissa, knowing that it wasn't up to her to give her baby a name.

'Mary has called her Sarah,' I replied. It was a special privilege given to the midwife assisting the birth to name the baby.

'That's lovely,' said Melissa and she looked away as the tears ran down her face. 'Can I see her?' she asked hopefully.

'Let me check with the charge nurse,' I replied as I replaced the chair near the wall.

An hour later, Therese, the charge nurse, brought Melissa her baby to see and to hold. She stayed and talked with her, answering more of her many, many questions. Melissa held Sarah, stroked her tiny fingers and lovingly touched her face. After an hour, Therese took Sarah back to the nursery.

The next morning, Melissa's parents came to take her home. She'd spent a restless night and looked very tired. The doctor had seen her, given her medication to dry up her breast milk, and asked that she return for a postnatal check-up in six weeks' time. By mid-morning she was ready to leave. If she was feeling sad as she walked through the postnatal ward past the other new mothers cooing at their babies, she certainly kept it to herself. Her face was expressionless. She paused at the nursery door and looked in to see if she could see Sarah. There were several babies tucked up tightly in their cots, but she couldn't tell which was her daughter.

News of a new baby up for adoption spread quickly through the maternity unit. Sarah was viewed by everyone from the cleaner to the matron. No one could resist gooing and gaaing at her, trying to get a reaction from her. Sarah's fragility and delicate features made everyone fall in love with her.

As the weeks went by, Sarah grew and started to take on her own personality. 'Give me a smile, you cheeky monkey,' teased Mary as she held Sarah on her lap. A big smile erupted on Sarah's face and her bright blue eyes shone with delight. This was quickly followed by a huge burp.

'That wasn't a real smile,' said Alice, coming into the nursery with a new baby. 'That was wind!'

Mary laughed. 'Get out of here!' she exclaimed. 'That was a smile, and that was especially for me!'

Sarah was the centre of attention in the nursery. At the time she was the only baby waiting for adoption and the midwives would take turns bathing, feeding and playing with her, singing to her and taking her for walks in the hospital pram around the park outside.

'Where's Mary?' asked the matron one morning. She looked outside to see Mary walking Sarah in the sunshine.

'Does she get any of her work done?' she asked Alice, who had come to stand beside her.

Alice laughed. 'Oh, yes. We all love Sarah, but we have to fight to look after her when Mary's around.'

Then one morning the charge sister, Trish, came into the nursery waving a letter. 'Sarah's new parents are coming next Wednesday to take her to her new home,' she announced.

I was holding Sarah at the time. Mary was on days off and I didn't have to fight anyone to feed Sarah this morning. 'That's good,' I remember thinking. Sarah had melted my heart and I always looked forward to going to work and hopefully being able to hold her, even for only a short time.

My mind wandered to Melissa and how hard it must have been for her to sign the adoption papers. Did she have any regrets? Since she'd left the hospital I had heard little tidbits on how she was getting on and how she'd gone away to visit relatives for a holiday.

We talked a lot about Michael and Sally, Sarah's new prospective parents, after that morning. We knew that Michael was a car salesman and Sally a receptionist, and that they had been trying to fall pregnant for three years before deciding to put their names on the adoption waiting list. Once they had met all the criteria the search had begun. They wanted a baby and not an older child, if possible. Sarah's photos had been shown to them and they had loved what they saw. Now they were coming to meet her.

On the day of Sally and Michael's visit, the nursery was full of midwives. Some were on duty, but others were on days off and just wanted to be there to see Sarah's new parents. Dressed in a simple white dress and a pink ribbon in her now growing hair, Sarah looked adorable. As Sally and Michael entered the nursery hand in hand, all eyes were upon them.

Sarah, who was being cuddled by Therese at the time, turned and smiled at them.

I looked at Sally and saw a tear run down her cheek. I felt a lump in my own throat and then also felt hot tears run.

Sally walked forward. 'Hello, Sarah,' she said 'I'm your new mummy.'

Michael also stepped forward and put his arms around his wife as she took Sarah in her arms. Applause erupted and all the midwives cheered, which startled Sarah and she began to cry.

'There, there,' said Sally soothingly, and soon the baby was smiling again.

Sally dressed Sarah in a frilly pink dress she and Michael had chosen for this special day. Each midwife then came to say goodbye to Sarah and to give Sally and Michael last-minute instructions.

'She likes to listen to Fleetwood Mac,' said Therese. 'You might have a little groover here.'

'Don't forget to read to her,' said Mary, standing close by. 'I will never forget you,' she whispered into Sarah's ear, and then hurriedly walked away.

'Sarah is very special to Mary,' explained Therese as she caught the puzzled look on Sally's face. 'She was there at Sarah's birth and was the midwife who named her.'

We followed a beaming Michael and Sally carrying Sarah as they walked down the stairs of the maternity unit and over to their car. Sarah looked like a little princess in her new pink dress and her little head was nestled close to Sally's shoulder.

'Take good care of her,' called Therese from the nursery window. Sally turned and waved.

'Can I take a photo of the three of you?' I asked Michael. 'One for the nursery photo board!'

He put his arm around Sally's waist and rested his other hand on Sarah's tiny little hand.

'We'd really like that,' said Sally.

They then carefully placed Sarah in her car restraint, climbed into their car, and with a beep from the horn, they were gone.

Weeks later we received the first of many letters and photos. They were all getting to know each other, and Sally and Michael were getting used to having less sleep than they usually had. They told us they'd decided to keep Sarah's name and not change it. The photos showed a smiling Sarah surrounded by soft, cuddly toys or being lovingly held by her parents.

Nearly twenty years on, I still think of Sarah. I ask myself: why did this little baby have such an impact on me? Was it my age and circumstances? I was married, yet childless, and just starting to think about having a family. Was it the timing of Sarah's birth during my midwifery training, and the experiences I gained looking after her? What was it about her? Why would someone totally unrelated to me in any way leave such a mark on my heart?

I find myself looking at twenty-year-old women today and wondering . . . could one of them be Sarah? What would I say to her if I ever got to meet her again? Would I ask her if she had been in contact with Melissa?

I hope that Sally and Michael have told Sarah how she was adopted and how special she is. Maybe it's true that angels come to earth as babies to teach us lessons. I think Sarah taught me, and all who met her, about love. She touched many lives and will never be forgotten.

The snow child

MEG JARVIS

When a woman confesses her intense desire to have a baby, how do you respond? I would like to be supportive, and respond in an understanding way, knowing that being able to talk might help. I try to listen well and hear exactly what the woman is saying to me.

There is always a fear of not being able to take away the pain. Will I be able to support her properly?

So, when Janice first spoke to me, I listened. She had spent five years trying to have a baby. She already knew how bad it could get, that feeling of wanting to have a child of your own, and then losing hope. Seeing others with children, watching pregnant women, feeling loss for something not yet realised. She had reached the depths of her despair. She had had one pregnancy some years before, and this had ended in a miscarriage. She was in her thirties and wanted a baby.

I could sense that she wanted to take control and try anything to conceive. She had looked at the moon charts, and taken medicines, berries and leaves. She was trying Clomid, the fertility drug, once again. Both she and Tom were seeing the specialists. Janice couldn't wait anymore.

How could I help her? I have heard women talk of seeing their babies before conception. Dreams of little ones playing in the garden. Faces that lift for a momentary glance somewhere near that window, and you were sure someone was there but when you looked, really looked, they were gone. No one talks of these images much.

There are stories about building children from wood or snow. At around the time Janice and Tom came to me, I remembered an old folk story from Russia called the 'The Snow Child'. In it, a woman and a man long for a child. They hear children playing in the snow nearby, laughing and shouting and making snowmen. The man and the woman, watching them, decide to make their own beautiful child out of snow. The snow child comes to life and joins them in their home. The man and the woman cherish her until the spring, when she melts and is gone again.

I remember in the story how the couple delighted in this child, and I told Janice the story. I tried to convey the beauty of the snow, the light on the child's face, the lips, the cheeks, the curve of the head and sweet curls. I thought Janice might like to make a 'snow child', but with clay. I told her where she could buy some, and I thought it might be best if, like in the story, she and Tom built their clay child together. Try to build a beautiful child, as they imagined their own baby to be.

'When you're finished, you could leave the clay child outside in the wind and the rain to melt away again into the elements, like some special gift you've now sown,' I said.

The clay child was made, but Janice kept her in their bedroom. Just a few weeks later, their own baby was conceived. Janice was joyful and smiling and looked very happy. The months and years of anxiety had disappeared. She began to grow and was knitting fine wool borders around soft blankets in preparation.

Their flesh creates anew that soft, sweet-smelling infant.

She still has some left-over clay somewhere, a memento of the time when she was waiting and nothing could ease her pain. It was a reminder that she did something to change how things were. I don't know if Tom knows where the clay is, and Janice didn't know either.

Perhaps Clare, their child, will find it and play with it with her soft, small hands.

When Janice reflects she says: 'How lucky are we? This divine child. So terribly, terribly lucky.'

Red lipstick

JACQUELINE JOHNSTONE

When I started my neonatal intensive care course in 1984, I was offered a mentor. This wasn't a structured arrangement, more an informal one, and students could choose if they wanted to participate. Faye was the epitome of what a neonatal nurse should be.

She had that kind, caring, gentle approach, and amazing skills and knowledge that I could only ever hope to achieve. On first meeting her, she appeared rather reserved, but once I got to know her, I found a very quick wit combined with a quirky sense of humour. She was always so beautifully groomed and was never without a touch of red lipstick to finish off her immaculate appearance.

Luckily for me, she happily took me under her wing. Once I began working with Faye, my life changed dramatically.

Even though I was the new kid on the block in an environment that scared the hell out of me, I covered up these feelings by allowing my vibrant personality to take over, and this allowed me to cope.

I was usually the type who felt comfortable making decisions, who stuck by my convictions, led the team, jumped in with both feet first, and was happy to bear any of the consequences. At no time did I intentionally want to be the leader, but it always seemed to be thrust upon me. I think it was because I was very outgoing and aired my opinions. Faye had many of the same thoughts and ideas, but as she was much quieter, many people didn't see that side of her personality. We often used to talk about how other people perceive you and how their ideas of where you should work and what you should be doing are indeed often very different from your own ideas.

I was a decision-maker, someone who had the courage of my convictions and managed change well, while Faye sat quietly in the background, coming up with the amazing ideas and fuelling us all.

During the course of our friendship, our professional relationship changed many times. After she was my mentor, we became colleagues, working together with tiny premature babies. The fun we had during some fairly scary and exhausting work experiences cemented our friendship. We always seemed to be working together when the unexpected twins, triplets or even quads arrived, and at the end of the shift we would laugh at some of the funny and unusual names that parents chose for their tiny babies.

A few years later, after we had both been working elsewhere around Australia – she in Queensland and me in Western Australia – we arrived back at the same hospital again. This time, however, I was the nurse manager and she the clinical midwife. In a role reversal, now the student was the mentor, but never at any time did I stop being in awe of her abilities and practices.

Most of the other staff felt the same way. Faye's holistic approach to caring and nurturing others triggers many memories for me. She was concerned, for instance, about how the myriad constant invasive procedures affected the tiny babies. She was determined to do something to reduce their agitation and pain.

One of the things she did was to place small cotton balls with a hint of lavender essential oil at the bottom of their cots to provide a calming environment. And lo and behold – they all calmed down, some even going to sleep!

The room also smelt fantastic for the staff. I'll never forget the look on the consultant's face that first morning during the ward round, when he opened the door to examine the babies and smelled the lavender wafting from every isolette. Initially he didn't like the idea of us using these oils, but was eventually won over when the data was presented to him and he saw how the babies reacted.

Now, whenever I smell lavender oil, I think of Faye, and of the way she taught me to occasionally sit quietly, relax and listen. She showed me how important it was to take time out, and now, whenever I have a massage, I remember her trying to instil in us all the need to care for ourselves.

Faye's role in the unit changed many times and she became, once again, the nurse educator. We worked together to help change and set up many new areas of practice for students, trained staff and parents in this neonatal unit.

As the neonatal educator she guided students to question practices that weren't evidence-based, and to look at the nursing care of these babies from the family's perspective. She taught them to involve the families in the care of, and decision-making about, the things they could do for their newborn.

So many groups of students were enthused about Faye's ideas. And just like in the movie *Dead Poets Society*, with Robin Williams as the teacher who dared to challenge his students, Faye was inspirational in nurturing their thoughts and beliefs. As testament to the respect they had for her teaching, the last group of students, on that final day in class, stood up on their chairs, held their hands over their hearts and repeated the words: 'Oh Captain, my Captain.'

No evaluation of that course was necessary. Their response said it all.

During a trip we had overseas lecturing to neonatal nurses in Hong Kong, Faye started to feel unwell. She lost a lot of weight and was exhausted most of the time. It happened very suddenly, and she thought it was just all the running around we had to do overseas. On our return, however, she eventually went to a doctor.

Faye was diagnosed with cancer.

Over the next few months, I watched my gentle, quiet, unassuming friend struggle with life. She had practised massage and alternative therapies for many years and was a very healthy person. Like most people, she couldn't understand how this had happened to her. She didn't smoke, and was a vegetarian. Her holistic belief system was challenged and her world turned upside down.

She worried about the effect her illness was having on her colleagues and her family, and whether she could finish the nursing education studies that she had started just prior to the onset of her illness. As always, she never wanted to let anyone down.

Finding it difficult to deal with what was happening to her, and not knowing how to fix it, she endeavoured to do what she always did – she set out to help other people.

Faye managed to complete a keepsake booklet for the parents of dying babies to help them overcome their own grief. Her lovely words that were written on the cover of the book are reproduced here:

> Be aware of the beauty of your child
> who leaves your side soon after you have met
> This loss removes the touch, but not the memories
> This silence is not an ending,
> but a voice of comfort and peace
>
> Remember your child like a flower to a garden
> Enjoy its beauty while it lasts
> Then let the memory linger in your heart
> When it fades the memories in this book will allow you
> to bring back the beauty of your loss

While Faye was having chemotherapy, we would talk about everything and anything. We would laugh till we hurt, remembering funny things we had done together. She loved to hear the gossip from work, and wanted to know of the babies that she had cared for in-between her days off work.

She nurtured my belief that having a clinical background was of great importance, and that I should return to this area of practice. Way back when she had first mentored me, she saw that my heart was in clinical practice, not management. We talked of this many times, just as we talked of what she would do when she was eventually able to return to work in the future. During the course of her treatment, after each session of chemotherapy, she would ring me and update me about her availability to come in and work. Initially it was just for one shift a week, but when she had a break between hospital sessions, she would do a few extra shifts. I never used to write her on the rosters in an official capacity, but just let her come in when she felt up to it. If she wanted to go home early, then that was okay too. She knew how much she could do, and what her weakened body could cope with each day, and it was her decision about where she would work in the nursery.

Throughout her illness, irrespective of how sick she was, Faye maintained her beautiful dignity and was always immaculate in her appearance. She came to work wearing the most amazing hats, and varying shades of red lipstick always adorned her lips.

Lipstick was one of her pleasures in life and even when very sick in hospital she managed to have it on. When I visited her the day before she died, she wanted to say goodbye. She knew we wouldn't meet again.

When I was leaving her hospital room and turned to wave my last goodbye, she smiled and I remember the colour clinging to her lips, a symbol of her enchanting and warm personality.

Her nickname, after all, had always been Lady Faye, and that was what she was.

As I approached the funeral chapel, afraid of what I might see, I was blind to everything else around me except the faces of those I had worked with for so many years. The chapel was large, bright and airy, despite being so crowded.

Outside it was a cold Melbourne day, but the sun was trying to shine through the large expanse of windows, straining to keep us all warm and to ignite in our hearts that feeling of warmth we had all felt for Faye. This congregation of people, many generations apart, wept openly. As they clung to each other for comfort, the most notable thing about them all was the varying shades of red lipstick every woman wore, the hues of scarlet, crimson and rose.

How can I describe what it was like? That sea of red lipstick was the ultimate mark of respect that Faye's friends and colleagues could show to the person who had taught them all so many things.

I've learned to stop occasionally and have that quiet time for myself, away from the frantic world all midwives work in. And so I go to the beach, walk with the sand squelching between my toes, and marvel at the amazing colours of the ocean. I look up to the skies, and I think of my friend.

I always carry my red lipstick in my handbag. Whenever I need that wee boost of spirit when I'm feeling down, out it comes to brighten my day, and I always think of Faye.

The other Florence

LEE PATTINSON

The obituary columns weren't Maria's usual choice of newspaper reading, but today she was checking the funeral arrangements made for a neighbour who had died. As she ran her finger down the fine print, she realised that her subconscious mind had registered another familiar surname on the way down: *Melinger* . . . Christian name: *Florence*.

Florence Melinger – not a name easily forgotten. Sister Florence Melinger. All those years ago. Twenty-five, in fact. She knew because that was exactly how old Ellen was. Born in the hospital where Sister Melinger had been on the administration staff.

Maria remembered that time so well. She'd been ready for discharge. Fourteen days they kept you in hospital back then, and she was finishing her packing, waiting for Don to come in and pick up her and the baby.

The nursery sister had already collected Ellen's 'going home' outfit, dressed her and carried her around the ward for the collective admiration of the other mums. Now the baby was back in her bassinette, waiting for her dad to arrive.

Maria had looked up at the sound of footsteps and seen Sister Melinger doing one of her 'swoops' to see that everything was at it should be. Nurse Atkins, the senior trainee midwife, hovered anxiously. Sister had an eagle eye and a sharp tongue. The nurse gestured towards Maria.

'Mrs Martin, Sister. She goes home today.'

'I have seen the discharge list, Nurse.'

Nurse Atkins blushed, threw an apologetic look at Maria and followed the ramrod-stiff back down the corridor.

Whew – hard and stiff as her uniform, that one! Probably looks the same on her whether she starched it or not. Nice, tender soul to have around if you weren't feeling well. Someone had mentioned that her first name was Florence, and had laughed: 'No relation to Florence Nightingale, I bet!'

Maria pulled out her sponge-bag, picked up her towel and headed for the ward bathroom for a last-minute brush-up. As she passed the small private room along the corridor, she thought about the poor mum in there. Nurses weren't supposed to talk about their patients, but it was surprising how news managed to filter along the hospital grapevine. Within a couple of hours of her arrival, everyone knew that Mrs James, mother of four boys, had given birth to two stillborn baby girls. And the patients knew that, as the days passed, the staff had become increasingly worried about Mrs James.

'Like a block of stone, she is. Hasn't moved a muscle

these three days. Just keeps her head turned towards the wall. Won't eat or drink or say a word, not even to her poor husband.'

That was one wardsmaid talking to another one, while they mopped the floor.

And Maria had heard two nurses talking in the sterilising room. 'Except for the fact that you can see her breathing, you'd think she was dead. Pat and I had to do a sponge bath and it was like handling a log of wood, only heavier. Sister says that if she's still not eating or drinking by tonight, she'll have to be tube-fed. That's one Rhyle's tube I wouldn't like to try passing!'

Now, as Maria pushed an ornamental comb into her hair and turned to return to the ward, she suddenly froze at the sound of a scornful voice coming from the slightly open door of Mrs James's room.

'. . . After all, you're not the first woman to lose a child!' It was Sister Melinger's voice. 'I fail to see what you think you'll accomplish lying here like a martyr, expecting to be waited on hand and foot! I suppose when you finally go home that poor husband of yours will be expected to pander to your selfishness – that's all it is, you know, selfishness! After all, they were his daughters too, or had you conveniently forgotten that?'

Whatever Sister Melinger had intended to say next was lost under the bitter, harsh gasp from Mrs James, and her furious 'Get out of here this minute, you . . . you *monster*!' Then the voice broke, and a storm of anguished weeping followed.

Maria stayed out of sight until she heard footsteps going down the corridor, then peeped out to confirm her identification of the speaker. After she heard the clang of the lift doors, she sought out Nurse Atkins at the nurses' station and asked if she could see Matron before leaving.

'She wouldn't have wanted her little speech overheard,' she thought grimly. 'Well, she'll soon find out it was!'

The nurse reached for the phone. 'Something wrong?' she asked worriedly. 'Anything I can do?'

Maria smiled in reassurance. 'Oh, nothing for you to worry about. Everyone on the ward has been absolutely marvellous. I've got no complaints about any of you.'

Relieved, Nurse Atkins spoke into the phone, and a moment later put it down and said: 'Take the lift down to the first floor and someone from Admin will meet you there.'

Ten minutes later, Maria was indignantly telling her story to the kind-faced matron. She was nervous, but determined to repeat what she had heard. There was a moment's silence when she finished.

'And what was Mrs James's reaction?' Matron asked calmly.

'What anyone might expect,' replied Maria firmly, a little taken aback. 'She ordered Sister Melinger to leave the room and called her a monster.'

Matron sighed, and said slowly: 'I suppose it probably seems that the matron of a hospital as big as this is kept so busy with paperwork that she loses track of more important things. However, I assure you that very little goes on that we don't know about.'

There was another pause before she continued quietly. 'In a way we resemble the army, and those of us who have had years in the profession know the value of discipline. To outsiders it may sometimes seem harsh, but we know from experience just how important it is. Which is why some of us are at times called on to perform a duty we personally find unpleasant – but we still do it.'

Maria interrupted Matron angrily. 'I can understand that – but what Sister Melinger did to that poor woman was both unnecessary and cruel!'

Matron was silent for another few seconds and then leaned forward. 'As you know, we avoid discussing individual patients but I think that in this case an exception can be made. You heard about Mrs James, I am sure – her tragic loss, her reaction . . .'

Maria nodded, and Matron continued. 'The one thing a midwife dreads in her career is a case of puerperal insanity. Postnatal depression is bad enough, but the other goes far beyond that. Mrs James was of great concern to all of us because of that real possibility. She had retreated from the world into a silent realm of her own, and she repulsed every attempt to break through the wall. Had she continued, there would have been little hope for her recovery. Can you imagine what that would have meant to her husband and four young sons?'

Maria shivered, then retorted: 'I don't see how Sister Melinger made things any easier for her, saying the things she did!'

Matron gave her a gentle smile. 'What did you tell me Mrs James's reaction was?'

Maria had no trouble recalling it. 'She called her a monster, and threw her out. When I passed, she was sobbing her heart out!'

'Exactly. And did you realise that that reaction was exactly what we had hoped for? We couldn't reach her with kindness, so harshness was our only answer. And Sister Melinger volunteered to try that route. Do you realise that Mrs James's words to Sister were literally the only ones she has spoken since the delivery?'

Maria still felt unconvinced. 'But Sister sounded as if she enjoyed doing it. She was so cold and unfeeling . . .'

'True discipline,' said Matron, 'embraces self-discipline, sometimes the hardest of all. Believe me, Sister Melinger was greatly distressed by the pain she had to inflict on Mrs James to shock her out of that silent, private world.'

Matron saw the scepticism on Maria's face and hesitated. 'You need proof, don't you?' she said. She rose, silently crossed to a door on the other side of her office, turned the knob with extreme care and beckoned. Maria walked over and peeped through the door.

She hardly recognised the proud, stiff figure of Sister Melinger as she sat, her face buried in her hands, filling the room with the sounds of uncontrollable, heartbroken weeping.

This event happened at Queen Victoria Hospital, Melbourne. I was the senior trainee midwifery student on the ward and the patient told me what had happened after she returned from seeing Matron to report the sister's actions.

Mrs James made progress, was discharged under doctor's watch and I never heard anything more during the rest of the year I was there.

Names have been changed, but the facts are as related.

Memorable mayhem

ELLIE McCUTCHEON

My first taste of midwifery was as a scared first-year 'junior night relief' (aka 'everybody's slave') nurse. It was, at first, a bitter taste. Barely six months out of preliminary training school, I worked in mid on weekends in our base hospital.

The weekend midwife, cranky and Irish, hated Australian doctors, nurses and hospitals. Verbal abuse from this unhappy harridan was commonplace, and occasionally, she flung forceps and bloodied swabs. One obstetrician, also Irish, told her to give me a fair go. She bullied on. I got more nervous than ever.

I put up with it for weeks, until I finally reached spitting point. In a voice I didn't recognise, I said that if she hated us so much, perhaps she should go home to Ireland.

'You must be homesick,' I added more gently. The following Saturday night when I trudged up the stairs, dreading another tirade, I found that a lovely, calm-natured redhead had taken her place. 'Irish' had given notice and gone home.

The replacement, Mardi, was an angel. With her, midwifery took on a whole new meaning and she inspired me to do mid training as soon as I could. When I was assisting her with deliveries, I felt I belonged. I became confident. Actually, arriving to have her own first baby over three years later, she became one of my very own early cases after graduating.

She wasn't so calm then, though – in fact, she was flustered, flushed and scared witless. Well, they say that most midwives make terrible mid patients! I would probably have been just as frightened and out of control, if I'd ever had children.

'Look, Mardi,' I said. 'What's all this? You were the calm, cool one who inspired me to do mid in the first place! Now look at you! Come on. Pull yourself together!'

She did.

Mardi was the perfect midwife, and I'm sure that all the women who were lucky enough to have her with them in labour never forgot her. I don't think any mother ever forgets the midwife who attends her, so we'd better all do our best.

There was a midwife on our floor whose husband was a policeman. His pay was poor, so Leanne worked full-time week-nights, even when pregnant. I admired her tenacity – she worked right to the very end. She was working, in fact, the night she started contracting, so she simply shaved herself, tested her wee, gave herself an enema, got the paperwork out, then called me to come in and take over. Leanne even had the foresight to put a hottie in the cot, ready for her baby. I call that dedication!

There'll always be that 'omnipotent' doctor or nurse who makes bald statements about when a baby will appear. There wouldn't be anything more daunting to a labouring mother than some 'prophet of doom' announcing that 'she isn't going to have the baby for hours yet' – even worse if the baby is in an occipito posterior position, causing unremitting backache and strong, pounding contractions every two minutes.

This prophesying is naive, as well as callous. Once the particular offender was gone, I'd whisper: 'Nobody can really predict *anything*, so we'll wait and see.'

It mightn't have sounded very ethical, but I hated seeing patients overwhelmed and fearful when this was supposed to be a joyous time. Having been given pain relief and positive reassurance, they often had a dramatic turnaround in proceedings, sometimes with breathtaking results.

One memorable morning, we had five babies in half an hour. (We had just two labour wards.) In the middle of this exciting ruckus, a primipara experiencing a POP (persistent occipito posterior) scenario suddenly wanted to just forget the pregnancy *and* the labour and go home. Who could blame her? Her doctor had just airily announced that she wouldn't deliver till about eleven o'clock that night.

When he had gone, I said this wasn't on. I got Jenny's husband to help with the mask and gave her some pethidine. Then I went next-door to move a newly delivered mother out of the labour ward so that I could scrub it down ready for the next one.

I'd been gone barely five minutes when Jenny's husband appeared, quite agitated. 'Ell!' he cried. 'She wants to push!' He ran back ahead of me.

I remember feeling some vindication for Jenny as I hurried back into the ward. She was sucking gas for all she was worth, really making the machine click, grunting through the mask. I checked and there was a decent bit of glossy black, curly-haired scalp. Reminding them how to puff through the contraction, I whizzed out for gloves, panting as I went.

Just then, her GP appeared. 'What's going on here?' he demanded pompously.

'David, you must be psychic. Jen's on view. I was just about to call you. I'll just get some gloves.'

'She can't be!' he retorted, glaring down his nose at me.

'Well,' I said. 'You go see for yourself, while I get gloves and a wheelchair.'

He was stunned to discover that I really knew what I was talking about, after all. It was too late for wheelchairs. We only had time to 'glove up' and Jenny was delivered in her bed. I'm not sure that David learned from the experience, though. He was never one to admit he got anything wrong. Fortunately, not all the doctors I worked with were like that! Most of them, I remember fondly.

One Saturday morning, Show Day, one of our SENs (State Enrolled Nurse), who was 36 weeks, called in to see me.

'Sis, I feel a little damp, like I'm leaking a bit. I was just going off to take my kids to the Show but thought

I'd better come here first. No contractions, just a bit of backache.'

I helped Jill up on to the labour ward bed and did a quick exam.

'Ooh! You're not going to the Show, Jill. You're fully dilated.'

She gasped. 'No! I can't be! I promised the kids! Their father's at work.'

I chuckled. 'Sorry, Jill. This baby is just about waving at us. Don't get up.'

I dialled the ward where her GP was doing rounds. He sprinted over and being one of those most rare cooperative types, helped me set up without being asked. Everything went smoothly and calmly. Five minutes later, there was this sweet-faced little girl lying on Jill's belly. I know it took Jill a bit to get over the shock of this swift arrival, especially when there'd been no real pain to announce it. The surprised looks on her kids' faces when I called them in from the waiting room were a treat.

Her husband thought we were 'having a lend of him' when we called him at work with the news.

Then there was a girl who came in off the street one Saturday. Connie was visiting in town. She was in labour – 36 weeks and booked for a Caesar back home, because of a breech with extended legs. I called in the duty doctor who was playing tennis on the hospital courts. He came and examined her at once. John was an experienced older GP who had seen and done it all.

I was stressed. I wearily contemplated having to get this girl organised for theatre despite being the only one on duty, with ten postnatals, their babies *and* two bed-ridden antenatals.

He saw my face, patted me on the arm and whispered, 'It's okay, Sis. If you'd just like to set up, I'll deliver her right here.'

Connie heard him. 'But my obstetrician, Mr Geeth, said I've got to have a Caesar!' she screeched.

John smiled. 'You're fully dilated now, my dear girl,' he said soothingly. 'Everything will be just fine.'

And it was. I watched in awe as this experienced old 'silvertail' skilfully extracted a small boy, breech with extended legs, in the twinkling of an eye.

The best-laid plans *can* go awry and the textbook descriptions of labour, delivery, and so on are usually just that; textbook descriptions that don't always match real life. Every patient is unique. There's no telling what might eventuate. We just have to listen to the patients and even if something sounds far-fetched or crazy, still take notice, and not fob them off.

In late 1969, the state was experiencing record births and I was a student midwife. A Greek woman in the five-bed antenatal ward of our frantically busy private mid unit in Melbourne called out to me as I went past with a delivery trolley.

'Seeester!' she squealed, her movements agitated. I went over to her.

She grabbed my hand, hard. 'I told the other one that there's something in the bed! She wouldn't listen!'

My heart racing, I pulled back the sheet, not sure what I would find. There, nestling comfortably between her thighs, was a plump, black-haired baby boy.

Something, all right!

Another night, I got the biggest shock ever. I was the only midwife on nights back at the base where I had trained. It was New Year's Day, 3 am.

'I thought we were going to have an early New Year's Day baby,' I said to my SEN.

'Oh, well. Four hours left! Anything can happen.'

I sent her off for an early breakfast. She had barely gone out the back door of the hospital, when the front doorbell clanged. Before I could do anything else, the lift clattered open on our floor and out leapt a very agitated woman in advanced second stage. She was clutching a little suitcase.

I knew Cassie well; I had delivered her twice before. She was one of those rarest of women who have a couple of contractions and then 'shell out' a baby with minimal fuss. I also knew that she was having twins this time and was staying in a flat opposite the hospital because of her past speedy performances. She was now 35 weeks.

She was hopping up and down, yelping: 'Oh, God! Oh, God!'

I scooped her into the wheelchair. We had a 50-yard dash up the passage to the labour ward. She had just got her backside on our fairly high bed and I was giving her a leg up, when I spied a little pink foot. I didn't have time to get her properly settled on the bed; in fact, she just had one leg anchored there before the owner of the said foot slithered out and I just managed to catch him. There was no time for the usual breech precautions, he was out! So much for allowing the head time to 'mould'! I swung her left leg up, clamped and cut his cord, and just had time to tag, wrap and hand him to his mother before there was a little blond head presenting and out came Twin Two, another small chap.

I think I only started breathing again once he, too, was warmly wrapped and on his mother's other arm. The placenta kindly followed without delay and it was all over; about three minutes from start to finish. Cassie hardly looked like she'd just had twins, and there was very little mess. It had all been extremely neat and tidy, but frighteningly fast. Feeling shaky with surging adrenalin, I dialled the GP's number. A sleepy, muffled voice answered.

'It's Sister G here,' I said. 'Um, Doctor, Cassie Jones has just had her twins.'

Before I could elaborate, he stuttered like a machine gun and roared, 'W-w-w-what the b-b-bloody hell! W-w-w-whaddya think you're playing at?'

But with that, suddenly fully awake, he realised who I was talking about and his tone softened. He apologised at once.

'S-s-sorry, Sis. Of course, she's one of those b-b-bloody quick women, isn't she! I'm on my way.'

By the time my SEN returned, Dr Cameron, with trousers and jumper over his pyjamas, was finishing checking Mum and babies. I'd also woken Cassie's deep-sleeping husband who hadn't even noticed she'd left. Nurse Jackson was gob-smacked. She just stood there with her mouth wide open and her pupils dilated with shock. She was speechless for ages. 'By the galore!' she finally managed to splutter. She had a few very strange turns of phrase in her vocabulary, I recall.

So, we got our New Year's Day babies (whose photo was on the front page of the local). An hour later, another mum arrived and so by 6 am we had three new babies in the nursery.

I practised mid for eighteen years, as well as neonatal nursing, and saw some strange, often awful, and sometimes funny things. Some things marked big changes in practice.

One day I was in theatre when a failed 'trial of labour' patient with a previous history of Caesarean section was about to be 'sectioned' again. As the obstetrician made the incision, opening the muscle layer, Mr James called me over.

'Hey, Sis. You'll never see anything like this again,' he said quietly. With another contraction, the previous longitudinal scar began to tear like fine tissue paper. What timing! Had it happened in the ward, the result probably would have been catastrophic for both mother and baby.

As it was, all went well because the obstetrician didn't dally and the theatre staff members were lightning fast at setting up, but there would be no more pregnancies after this one.

It was a clear demonstration as to why all incisions are, these days, made in the lower uterine segment.

Later, a friend had a huge bleed, after having undiagnosed 28-week twins, and on the first night was having a blood transfusion. She was supposedly well-sedated because it had been a horrific day, with the smallest twin collapsing frequently. The girl on night duty went in with her torch, to check on her and do blood obs, but found her gone. She followed a trail of dots of blood. The patient, Annie, had somehow managed to chew through her IV tubing (she must have had awfully sharp teeth) and staggered off to the toilet in her sleep. We never told Annie what happened that night; she would have been so mortified.

Another first-day Caesar patient actually walked out of the hospital, unnoticed, in the middle of the night and the police found her miles away, in her short, green, backless hospital gown, with her bare bottom showing. She was heading for home, still conscientiously carrying her IV bottle.

I was never known for my ball-handling skills, but one day I was naively trying to encourage a mum-to-be not to push just yet, as we were trying to get our gloves on at least. But naturally this fell on deaf ears – you can't tell a woman giving birth not to push. Anyway, she was pretty agitated and scared because she was only 28 weeks. I was all of six weeks into my mid training then. All of a sudden, she gave a sharp, loud grunt from her throat and expelled a 1000-gram baby. He sailed through the air past my face and I miraculously managed to mark him like you'd mark a football. He had carroty red, downy hair and big, beady, dark blue eyes. I'd love to meet him now! He would be 35 years old!

Another day my mid super, Bessie, and I were assisting our favourite obstetrician with a difficult birth. The labour had been exceptionally exhausting for this mother of four. When the long, thin boy was finally born, he was flat and pale, not breathing and his heart was merely fluttering. Bessie and I are both Christians and we felt compelled to start praying for help as we worked on this scrawny, lifeless little bloke.

There wasn't much in the way of neonatal resuscitation equipment back then; all we had was a heat lamp, the oxygen catheter and the good old 'frog breathing' technique. It took about twenty minutes, but finally he started breathing on his own. Our obstetrician, an agnostic, quietly said: 'You know, I don't believe in God, but now I have to really wonder, after seeing you two at work.'

The baby survived well and has grown up to become a fine young man and a wonderful ambassador for Australia in his chosen area of expertise.

I started midwifery in 1969, so I have witnessed other dramatic changes in the care of mothers and babies. Then, in our unit in Melbourne, most mothers stayed in hospital for at least seven days; some obstetricians even kept patients in for up to fourteen days. One female obstetrician insisted that hers couldn't even get up to shower for seven days! We tended to turn a blind eye to these mums sneaking out of bed for a shower when Dr Green was gone. En-suite bathrooms were so practical.

But we were still doing perineal rounds and wash-downs four-hourly around the clock on everyone with sutures. Fathers didn't come into the labour ward, there was no rooming-in, and all term babies were fed strictly four-hourly. The nursery staff did the 1 am feed so that the mothers got a good rest. It was fun and games, two people trying to feed 30 or 40 hungry babies!

A year later, when I returned to my old stamping ground in the country, things were more relaxed than in Melbourne. Most fathers were there for the birth, there was rooming-in if desired and demand feeding. There were very few wash-downs, and the fathers had an extra hour of visiting time every evening. They were encouraged to collect their babies from the nursery trolley (which held nine babies) and take them to the room for private time. We even sent them out for a night on the town, the night before discharge. Of course, the pendulum of change always seems to swing too far in the opposite direction and I wonder if new mothers get enough rest and TLC these days before they're back home.

I've been out of midwifery for eighteen years now. Back problems prevent me from returning. Though midwives are desperately needed all around the country, I know I couldn't manage, but every time I meet a pregnant woman, I have huge twinges of longing for the old times when I was happiest practising midwifery and neonatology. I can almost smell those aromas peculiar to labour and birth.

Of course, I can't remember every single baby I helped care for, but to me, they are all my family and there are many that I still know about. I am almost as proud of them as I would be if they were my own.

GLOSSARY

Alligators – An instrument used for performing artificial rupture of the amniotic sac membranes. See also **ARM** and **rupture of membranes.**

Ambubag – A bag and mask used to ventilate babies who require resuscitation.

Amnihook – A device used for performing artificial rupture of membranes.

Antenatal – Before birth.

APH (antepartum haemorrhage) – When bleeding occurs from the birth canal after 24 weeks of pregnancy and before the birth of the baby.

Apgar score – A scoring system devised by Dr Virginia Apgar to assess the condition of a baby during its first few minutes of life.

ARM – Artificial rupture of membranes.

Bagged – When oxygen is administered to a baby via a mask.

Breech – When the baby is in a longitudinal position with the buttocks lying lowermost in the uterus and the head in the upper part of the uterus.

Caesarean section – Surgical removal of the baby and placenta via the woman's abdomen. Also known as LUSCS, or lower uterine segment caesarean section.

Cerebral oedema – An excess of fluid accumulated in the brain.

Cervix – The neck or the lower part of the uterus, which is about 2.5 centimetres long and opens into the vagina.

Colostrum – The yellowish fluid secreted by the breasts during pregnancy and before the beginning of lactation.

Cord prolapse – When the membranes of the amniotic sac have ruptured and the umbilical cord descends below the presenting part of the baby.

CTG (cardiotocography) machine – Equipment to monitor the foetal heart rate before birth.

Curette – A surgical procedure that expands the opening of the uterus to allow removal of contents of the uterus. Also known as D&C, dilatation and curettage.

Depo injections – A form of contraception given by injection at three-monthly intervals. Also known as Depo-provera.

Dilation – The measurement used to identify the dilatation of the cervix during the first stage of labour. The cervix dilates from closed to 10 centimetres.

Dyspareunia – Difficult or painful intercourse.

EBM – Expressed breast milk.

Epidural – An injection of a local analgesic administered into the epidural space, situated in the lower part of the spine, to provide pain relief during childbirth and/or during and after surgery.

Episiotomy – An incision made into the perineum during birth.

FDIU – Foetal death in utero.

Foetal bradycardia – Slowing of the baby's heart rate below 110 beats per minute during pregnancy or prior to birth.

Foetal tachycardia – Increase in the baby's heart rate above 160 beats per minute during pregnancy or prior to birth.

Forceps – Surgical instruments with two blades used in obstetrics for extracting the baby's head from the birth canal.

Frog breathing – An old method used for resuscitating a baby which, by manually opening and closing the baby's mouth and nasal passages, creates a build-up of oxygen pressure in the baby's lungs and stimulates respiration.

Fundus – The top of the uterus.

Gavage feeding – When fluids are fed to a baby through a tube inserted into its stomach via the mouth or nose.

Gravida – A pregnant woman.

Hartmanns – An intravenous fluid.

Hb (haemoglobin) – A pigment contained in the red blood cells which transports oxygen to the tissues.

Iliac fossa – A large shallow depression forming much of the inner surface of the large hip bone.

Induction of labour – Intervention to stimulate uterine contractions before the onset of spontaneous labour.

Infusion pump – A machine that is used to control the flow of intravenous fluid into the body.

Lactation – The secretion of milk by the breasts.

Liquor – The fluid that surrounds the baby in the amniotic sac.

Lotus birth – Following birth the umbilical cord is not cut so that the baby and placenta remain attached until separation of the cord occurs naturally, usually between three to ten days following birth.

Meconium – A soft greenish-black viscid substance that accumulates in the baby's bowel from the 16th week of intra-uterine life, and is usually passed during the first few days of life. Passing of meconium during labour can indicate that the baby is distressed.

Membranes – These cover the baby's side of the placenta and form the amniotic sac, which contains the baby and the amniotic fluid.

Moro reflex – Otherwise known as the 'embrace' or 'startle' reflex where the baby extends their arms in response to sudden movement or noise.

Moulding – Alteration to the shape of the baby's head during labour.

MRI – Magnetic Resonance Imaging, a diagnostic imaging method used by radiologists to view internal body structures in much greater detail than ultrasound or x-ray.

Neonatal – Pertaining to the newborn child.

Neonatology – A speciality of medicine that deals with disorders of the newborn child.

Nipple shield – A soft device applied over the nipple to facilitate breast feeding.

Obs – Observations on a woman and/or her baby as

required. These can include temperature, pulse, blood pressure and breathing rate.

Oxygen saturation – The amount of oxygen bound to the red blood cells.

Oxytocic – A term applied to any drug that stimulates the uterus in order to induce or accelerate labour. See also **oxytocin.**

Oxytocin – The natural hormone that stimulates contraction of the uterus. Oxytocin can be produced synthetically, e.g. Syntocinon.

Palpation – A systematic examination of the abdomen by touch during pregnancy and labour.

Pelvimetry – Measurement of the size of the pelvis performed either clinically or by radiography.

Perineum – The muscular pyramid between the lower third of the vagina anteriorly and the anal canal posteriorly, and the lower protruding pelvic bones (ischial tuberosities) laterally.

Placenta muncher – A machine used in some birthing units to dispose of the placenta following birth.

Postnatal – After birth.

Posterior position – The baby is positioned with head down and back between the mother's spine and hip bone. Also known as occipito posterior position. Persistent occipito posterior (POP) occurs when the baby does not turn during labour.

Prolapse – Refers to the descent of one or more of the pelvic structures due to weakness of the pelvic floor. The uterus, vaginal walls, bladder or rectum may be involved.

Prostaglandin gel – A synthetic gel used to ripen the cervix and induce labour.

Pudendal block – An injection of local anaesthetic administered around the pudendal nerve used as pain relief prior to vaginal operative births.

Primigravida – A woman having her first baby. Also known as primipara.

Puerperal insanity – A rare and severe episode of post-natal depression.

Ringers – An old term used for an intravenous solution.

Rupture of membranes – Occurs when the amniotic sac tears or is punctured, either spontaneously or artificially. Also known as ROM.

Scalp probe – An electrode that is applied to the baby's head and connected to a cardiotocography machine to record the baby's heart rate.

Show – A term used to denote the blood-stained discharge at the onset of labour that comes from the cervical canal plug.

Shoulder dystocia – A rare complication occurring after birth of the baby's head, in which the shoulders fail to rotate, descend and birth.

Stages of labour – First stage: Used to describe labour from the onset of regular painful contractions, during which time the cervix thins and becomes fully dilated. Second stage: Refers to labour from the time the cervix is fully dilated until the baby is born. Third stage: The time from the birth of the baby until the placenta has been birthed. Physiological third stage involves a 'hands off' approach whereby separation and birth of the placenta and membranes occurs spontaneously; active management involves the administration of a synthetic oxytocic drug, and the birth attendant assists with the delivery of the placenta and membranes.

Syntocinon – Synthetic oxytocin administered intravenously to induce or augment labour.

Third-degree tear – A complete tear extending through the whole of the perineal body, through the anal sphincter and into the rectum.

Transition – The transitional period between the dilation, or first stage of labour, and the time when active maternal pushing efforts begin.

Transverse lie – When the longitudinal axis of the baby lies across the mother's uterus.

Tympanic – Refers to a section of the ear. A tympanic temperature measurement is used to measure the temperature of children and adults.

Ventouse extraction – When a baby is delivered by vacuum suction. A cup is applied to the baby's scalp, and suction and gentle traction are used in conjunction with maternal pushing to draw the baby out of the vagina.

Vernix – The greasy white substance that covers the baby in utero.

ABOUT THE CONTRIBUTORS

Nola Aicken is a Lecturer in Midwifery who works within the academic and clinical environments of La Trobe University and the Bendigo Health Care Group. She has practiced as a midwife for many years, and is passionate about maintaining a rural focus for regional and rural midwives. Her PhD studies will explore the issues for midwives in regional Victoria.

Sue Baker is a Midwife and Maternal and Child Health Nurse with almost twenty years' experience. She is passionate about working with families and believes that midwives and child health nurses are privileged to be invited into other people's lives. She lives and works in country Victoria.

Robin Barker is a registered Nurse, Midwife and Child

and Family Health Nurse. She is the author of *Baby Love*, *The Mighty Toddler* and *Baby and Toddler Meals*.

Dianne Boshammer hails from the western Queensland town of Brigalow. After graduating from Chinchilla High School she began midwifery studies at the Mother's Hospital in Toowoomba, which she completed in 1986. She has two fabulous teenage daughters and currently lives and works in Mudgee, New South Wales, at the local Mudgee District Hospital.

Christine Croyden began nursing at seventeen, travelled extensively and worked in the UK and France. She returned to Australia in 1986 to train as a midwife and later left the profession to study arts. She has three children and lives in Melbourne, where she now writes full time. Her work has been published in Australia and overseas.

Shona Davidson emigrated from her native Scotland in 1990 and since then has travelled around Australia working in midwifery, neonatal ICU and neonatal transport. She is currently working in adult ICU. A true 'Scots-tralian', her time is spent exploring the bush by foot, bicycle and 4WD. This is her first published story.

Susan Demoray left nursing for other passions – writing, children and family. A graduate in literature and philosophy, she has had a non-fiction book published and has writing credits in the corporate sector, film, radio and the web. Currently, Susan works in music promotion and markets her quirky rock industry novella for women.

Maree Eggleston works in delivery suite and parent education, and is currently completing a Diploma of Arts (Professional Writing and Editing). This is the third short story she has had published. She is also writing a tell-nearly-all novel about surviving General Nurse Training and the 1970s.

Linda Fabb has worked as a midwife in community and hospital settings. She helped organise the Australian Nursing Journal 1996 short story competition, which resulted in publication of *From the Heart: True stories by Australian nurses*. She lives an idyllic life with her partner and two children in the Yarra Valley, and aims to walk lightly on the earth.

Monica Feder moved to the remote area of the West Wimmera Shire on completion of her nursing studies at the Royal Melbourne Hospital in 1990. She is married to Mark and they live and work on a farming property with their children, Madeline and Adam.

Kate Field is a midwife living in rural Victoria with her husband and four children. She is currently studying a Master of Nursing. Her passions include midwifery, horse riding, travelling and writing. In the future she hopes to move to the coast and travel to Africa and South America.

Heather Harris graduated as a midwife in 1970 and has worked in various maternity settings. After completing her Masters degree she served as a midwife in West Africa and Sri Lanka with Medecins Sans Frontières. She is an educator and has produced three videos which are distributed globally. She has two grown children.

Bronni Hawksworth is a Kiwi nurse who completed her Graduate Diploma in Midwifery in Australia. After gaining twelve months experience in private and public hospitals, she left to have her children at home and establish a private practice in the hills of the Yarra Valley.

Lyn Hoffman has worked in the Shepparton area for many years in both the District Nursing Service and local hospitals. She is currently employed at Goulburn Valley Health as a Domiciliary Midwife and enjoys the varied challenges of nursing out in the community. Lyn is married with two adult children.

Laraine Hood has been a midwife for seven years. She recently completed a Masters degree in Midwifery at Curtin University, and moved to Loose Goose Chalets in Nannup, Western Australia, with the dream of creating a midwifery retreat and education centre in the bush.

Meg Jarvis graduated as an Anthroposophical Nurse, having studied medicinal plants, and later went on to become a full-time midwife. She is passionate about midwifery, and also paints women, birth, midwives and their journeys. She is married with three sons.

Jacqueline Johnstone is currently a Clinical Midwifery Educator. Her formal qualifications include Midwifery, Neonatology, Lactation Consultancy and Education. She has worked in a variety of positions ranging from developing a neonatal program for midwives in the Philippines, to flight nurse for the Royal Flying Doctor Service in Western Australia.

Olivia Langley worked in maternal and child health centres for many years, continuing to work part-time when she married Kevin and had two children. She and Kevin are now retired and live in Gippsland, Victoria. Olivia enjoys watching her three grandchildren grow up, and occasionally babysits.

Genevieve Lilley has been a midwife for five years. Previous, less emotionally stimulating jobs include general nurse and philosophy tutor. She now also works as a women's health nurse and family planning nurse.

Sandra Linklater has more than 25 years' experience in child and family health. She has nursed mothers and babies from many religious, cultural and social backgrounds. Using her extensive knowledge, Sandra wrote and produced two CDs, *Baby's First Six Weeks* and *Toddler Magic*.

Ellie McCutcheon is a handspinner, gardener, sheep-breeder, Professional Writing and Editing student, disability support tutor, aged care administration volunteer, newsletter editor and non-fiction writer. The sights, sounds and unique odours of mothers and neonates remain strong memories, and she still feels midwifery's spell on meeting pregnant women.

Brooke McReynolds was born on a farm in Kansas and now lives in Australia. She has worked as an obstetric nurse, a midwife, and in the area of public health. Her workplaces have included hospitals, prisons and clinics.

A. E. Moates started nursing in Queensland in the early 1980s before travelling and working overseas. She currently resides in Victoria, where she gained her midwifery and maternal and child health credentials. Over the years she has specialised in many areas but her focus has been on the care of infants, young children and their families. She is also interested in history and ethics.

Shannon Morris is part of the Canberra Midwifery Program team and occasionally works independently for women birthing at home. She is a perpetual student and is currently completing her Masters in Midwifery with a project exploring fear around birth. She is married and has a daughter, Lily, who was born at home.

Carol Morton is an English-trained Registered Nurse and Midwife who has more than 25 years' experience in general nursing, midwifery and neonatal intensive care. She is married with two teenage children.

Prue O'Halloran has worked across many areas of nursing throughout her career and never returned to nursing in the city. She encourages young RNs to seek out and embrace the challenges that can be found by working with Aboriginal communities, because the experience can be life-changing.

Lee Pattinson was a nurse at Prince Henry Hospital in Melbourne before training to become a midwife at Queen Victoria Hospital. She has worked extensively in infant welfare, practising mostly in regional areas, and for many years had a weekly column in *New Idea* magazine. She has three grandchildren and two great-grandchildren, with another on the way.

Jennifer Richmond started nursing in the days of starched aprons and still works part-time in sub-acute care. She also has written and collaborated on a number of nursing publications, including the acclaimed *Unique and Ordinary*. Her first long work of fiction will be published in 2005.

Jan Robinson runs a clinical practice in southern Sydney and limits her annual client load to twenty to maintain a balance of quality midwifery care and quality education services. Jan's formal qualificaions include a Master of Midwifery, Bachelor of Applied Science and Dip Nurse Ed. She is a Fellow and Accredited Independently Practising Midwife with the Australian College of Midwives.

Jan Roughley works as a Maternal and Child Health Nurse in Melbourne, and has twenty years' experience in nursing. Her qualifications include general nursing, midwifery, child, family and community health, and lactation consultant. She has a Graduate Diploma in Advanced Nursing. Of particular interest to her is assisting clients from culturally diverse backgrounds.

Helen Sandner is a midwife consultant working in private practice. She is a member of the Maternity Coalition and Midwives In Private Practice, and a Fellow of the Australian College of Midwives. Helen also enjoys her involvement as a mentor and sessional lecturer of undergraduate and postgraduate midwifery students.

Annie Sprague is an independent midwife who has attended births at home and in hospital for more than twenty years. Her strong interest in the use of water during childbirth led her to research and write *Water Labour, Water Birth*, a guide aimed at complementing good midwifery practice.

Judy Thomson lived overseas for several years before starting nursing as a mature age student at the Royal Adelaide Hospital. She then became a midwife at the Queen Victoria Hospital. For many years she was the Midwifery Nurse Educator in Broken Hill, and now works in health promotion in Port Macquarie.

Susan Timpani has worked as a nurse in hospices, labour wards and in the community. From the poverty of India to the isolation of Papua New Guinea and the special needs of Adelaide's Aboriginal community, her experiences have been diverse. She is married with four children and is currently writing a novel.

Marie Treloar was the recipient of the Irving Buzzard Midwifery Prize for 2003. She is one of the key founders of The Highlands Foundation, which is dedicated to improving the health of women and children in the remote highlands of Papua New Guinea. Marie is currently pursuing a Masters in Public Health (International Health Stream) at Melbourne University.

Joanne Vine was born in England in 1966 and immigrated to Australia with her family when she was five years old. She lives in a small country town and when she is not looking after her husband and three children, she is a midwife in a large regional hospital.

ACKNOWLEDGEMENTS

The following people and organisations have given their time, support and encouragement. We're grateful for their input and enthusiasm:

Australian College of Midwives Inc., with special thanks to the North Central Victorian Branch.

Members of the Midwives, Miracles and Mayhem project team: Marie Treloar, midwife, Bendigo Health Care Group; Nola Aicken, Lecturer in Midwifery, La Trobe University, Bendigo; and Helen Sandner, midwife consultant. We offer special thanks to Nola and Helen for compiling the glossary.

The Australasian Medical Writers Association for the 2003 AMWA award, which allowed Amanda to attend the ACMI conference in Perth and commission stories directly from midwives.

Anne Donald for designing publicity material. Sue Alexander, Linda Fabb, Robin Barker and Marea

Vidovich for helping us to spread the word to midwives.

Jill Illiffe and Krista McClelland at the Federal office of the Australian Nursing Foundation for promoting the project to ANF members via the *Australian Nursing Journal* and the ANF national website.

Stella Glorie of the Victorian Writers' Centre for advertising the project through State Writers' Centres.

Jane Thompson, midwife and musician, for inspiration and encouragement.

Barbara Vernon, ACMI executive officer for valuable background information.

We had lots of help from our friends and families, who provided childcare, meals and editorial feedback: Greg Flynn, David Dore, Sophie Risstrom, Carmel Dick, Olivia Tattam, Emma Tattam and the Cowie family in Castlemaine.

Finally, to all the midwives who found the time, energy and creativity to write about their working lives, thank you for trusting us with your stories.